Contents

KU-544-369

Part 1: Triathlon Basics

3

Part 2: Equipment

19

Part 3: Swim

51

Part 4: Bike

79

Part 5: Run

Part 6: Transition

Part 7: Strength Training and Stretching

Part 8: Triathlon Training Programs

Part 9: Race Day

Glossary

Index

Introduction

You might want to get into triathlons because you've heard your coworkers talk about their experiences and it sounds like fun. You might want to get in shape. You might have seen the Ironman broadcast on television and marveled at the suffering that the athletes were willing to put themselves through in the Hawaiian lava fields. You might already have a couple triathlons under your belt but you're ready to take it to the next level. Whatever your reason, this book is for you!

Triathlon is more than just a sport—it is a journey of self-discovery, determination, and endurance. Be prepared to push yourself, maybe harder than you've pushed yourself physically or mentally in the past. We will be with you every step of the way.

Maybe you're not quite sure what a triathlon is. The standard triathlon consists of swimming, biking, and running, almost always in that order. The swim is usually the shortest stage and the bike the longest. The glue that holds each sport together is called *transition*. You'll practice this, just like the other three disciplines, and learn to efficiently drop the gear that you no longer need, and grab what you need going forward. Swim, transition, bike, transition, run ... that's it!

Anyone can get involved in this growing sport; there are no physical or mental prerequisites. Even if you don't know how to do one of the three sports, it's not too late to start. Nobody is born with the ability to swim, ride, or run—we all learn these skills. If you're already comfortable with any or all of the three disciplines, you've got that much of a head start. Now we will work on putting them all together.

Many triathletes who come to us have already done a TRI or two but felt like they were ill prepared for the event. They suffered through and made it to the finish line, but they want to become more efficient at a sport to which they're newly addicted. Is this you? If so, this book will get you focused!

Was this book a gift from a well-meaning friend or relative? Are you standing in a bookstore wondering if this is something you should even attempt? Everyone can think of a list of reasons that they can't do something ...

> *I just don't have the time.*
>
> *Swimming scares me.*
>
> *I haven't run since high school.*

You can do this! You just need to decide: I *will* do this.

Bill Bell and other triathletes have competed in the Ironman World Championship into their eighties. Dick Hoyt has propelled his paraplegic son, Rick, through that same race multiple times (as well as through 1,000 other endurance events). If you have an "I can't" reason, would you be willing to put it up against theirs?

The only requirements for this sport are determination, desire, and attitude. You have what it takes. Dig down and decide that you are going to accomplish this goal. We'll supply the inspiration and explanation. Let's get started!

Acknowledgments

Steve and Colin would both like to thank their families, friends, and coaches for all their support and understanding throughout their triathlon journey. They'd especially like to acknowledge Paul Huddle, Paula Newby-Fraser, Roch Frey, and Bob Babbitt for imparting some of their boundless knowledge about the sport.

Additionally, thanks to those who contributed to this book project with your photo support: Jay Prasuhn, 2XU, Aqua Sphere, MarathonFoto, and Nytro Multisport.

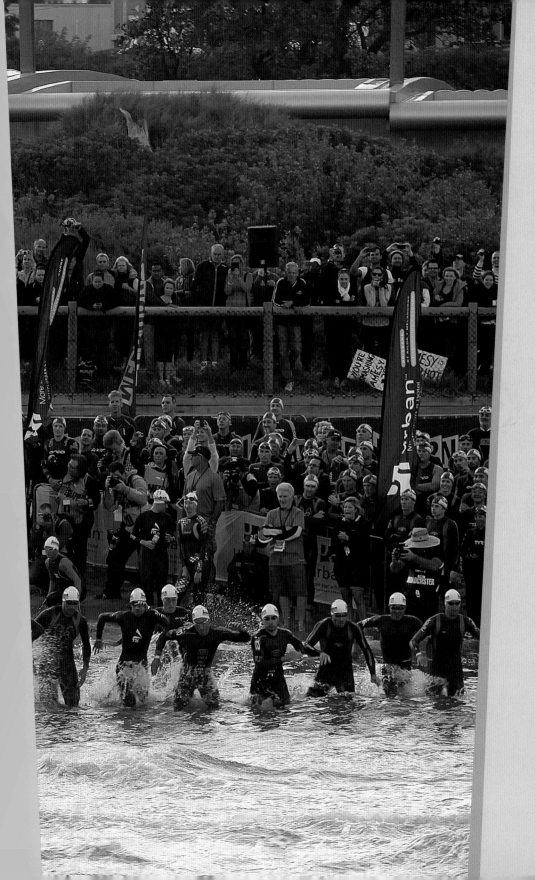

Triathlon Basics

To many people, participating in a triathlon sounds like a crazy endeavor. Swimming, biking, and running long distances, all in succession? Why would anyone do this? Answers to that question vary as much as individual personalities do. Some participants like that triathlons, often called TRI, offer a new way to push the mind and body. Others enjoy the camaraderie offered by races and local TRI clubs. Many see it as a great way to get fit and lose some weight. Whatever your reason, the TRI world will welcome you with open arms and complete encouragement.

Before you get started on your triathlon journey, there are a few basics you need to know. This part will provide some background on triathlons and help you choose the type of TRI event that's best for you.

What Is a Triathlon?

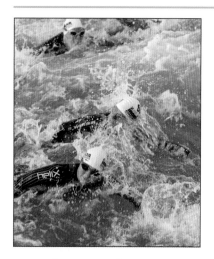 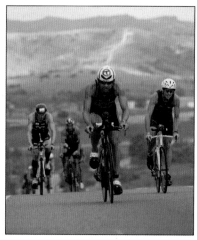 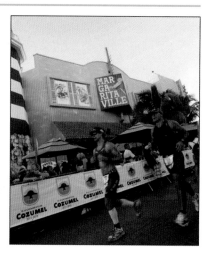

Any multi-stage endurance event in which three different sports are completed consecutively can be considered a triathlon. This book focuses on the standard triathlon, which combines swimming, biking, and running. The distance of each stage can vary, as can the total distance of the event; however, there are some standard triathlon distances that are used around the world.

Common Triathlon Distances

	Super-Sprint	Sprint	Olympic	Half-Ironman	Ironman
Swim	0.2–0.3 miles (300–500 m)	0.25–0.5 miles (375–750 m)	0.9 miles (1.5 km)	1.2 miles (1.9 km)	2.4 miles (3.86 km)
Bike	6–10 miles (10–16 km)	6.2–13.2 miles (10–22 km)	24.8 miles (40 km)	56 miles (90 km)	112 miles (180.25 km)
Run	0.5–2 miles (1–3 km)	2–3.1 miles (3–5 km)	6.2 miles (10 km)	13.1 miles (21.1 km)	26.2 miles (42.2 km)
Total	About 7 miles (15 km)	About 10 miles (20 km)	31.9 miles (51.5 km)	70.3 miles (113 km)	140.6 miles (226 km)

Although these are common triathlon distances, TRI events can be shorter (6 miles or less) or much longer. For those with extreme commitment and endurance, there are ultratriathlons that are double the distance of the Ironman or more!

The History of Triathlon

The first triathlon on record was held in San Diego (Mission Bay), California, in 1974. Forty-six participants, both males and females, took part in a 6-mile run, a 5-mile bike, and a 500-meter swim.

U.S. Navy Commander John Collins, one of the athletes who raced that day, helped take the sport to the next level. He brought the triathlon concept to Hawaii and in 1978 combined three of Oahu's previously established endurance events—the Waikiki Rough Water Swim, the Around-Oahu Bike Ride, and the Honolulu Marathon—into one 140.6-mile race: the Ironman.

Two years later, ABC's *Wide World of Sports* televised the event. People across the globe were inspired and overwhelmed with emotion as they watched the Ironman athletes truly put their bodies to the ultimate challenge. Participation and interest for triathlons of all distances have grown exponentially since that televised moment.

Triathlon Milestones

1974 The San Diego Track Club Newsletter advertised its new race with a headline reading, "Run, Cycle, Swim: Triathlon set for 25th of September," using the word *triathlon* for the first time in the modern sense.

1978 Fifteen men started the first Ironman; twelve finished. Gordon Haller became the first Ironman champion, winning the race in 11 hours, 46 minutes, 58 seconds.

1982 Second-place finisher Julie Moss' unforgettable crawl to the Ironman finish line shown on ABC's *Wide World of Sports* and inspired many to take up triathlon.

The Torrey Pines Triathlon, won by Dave Scott, was both the first United States Triathlon Series event and the first triathlon to offer prize money.

1983 Spin-offs of the San Diego Track Club Newsletter called "Triathlon," and "Tri-Athlete," founded by William Katovsky, became the first triathlon publications.

1984 Timex Corporation created the "Triathlon" watch and then joined with Ironman organizers to use the name "Ironman."

1985 Triathlon sparked a cross-training fitness boom. Nike featured pro triathlete Joann Ernst in national ad campaigns.

1993 Triathlon was approved for inclusion at the 1995 Pan Am Games in Mar del Plata, Argentina.

1994 The first Goodwill Games Triathlon was held in St. Petersburg, Russia.

1997 The United States Olympic Committee (USOC) officially recognized USA Triathlon as an Olympic Sport Organization.

2000 Triathlon debuted as an Olympic sport in Sydney, Australia.

2013 Ironman celebrated its thirty-fifth anniversary in Kona, Hawaii.

Health and Fitness Benefits

TRI is an excellent sport for improving health and fitness. Through training and competition, your body adapts to gradually increased workloads, which improves your cardio-respiratory function. In addition, you build more muscle throughout your body and lose fat. The increase in muscle tone contributes to a higher resting metabolic rate. In other words, you burn more calories even when you're not doing anything. When you train for a triathlon, the focus on endurance coupled with power and strength components (e.g., resistance training and interval training) allow for balanced conditioning.

Beyond simply feeling great, some of the potential health benefits of TRI include:

- Lower LDL (bad) cholesterol levels in the blood
- Higher HDL (good) cholesterol levels in the blood
- Reduced chance of strokes and heart attacks
- Lower blood pressure
- Reduced chance of diabetes
- Better overall body composition
- Stronger bones (from weight-bearing exercise)

The Power of Cross-Training

Cross-training simply means that you include a variety of exercises in your fitness program. TRI, by nature, employs this principle. Two major benefits of cross-training are the reduction in boredom and the ability to manage injuries. When you train for a triathlon, you have to train for all three sports. This keeps your workouts fresh and engaging, and prevents you from becoming burned out on one type of exercise. As a result, the number of people who keep up with their workout regimen increases dramatically. Fitness becomes a lifestyle and no longer a chore. Your mindset begins to shift from needing to psych yourself up for a workout to not even considering skipping training.

Even if you're feeling engaged and motivated by your workouts, an injury can be a major setback. If you do experience an injury, it's possible to employ cross-training principles to aid in your recovery. With cross-training, you usually won't have to give up your entire fitness program; you may be able to modify or substitute activities. For example, if your knee has been aching from running increased distances, you can back off of running while increasing your swim or biking distances. This gives your body time to recover while maintaining your level of cardiovascular conditioning.

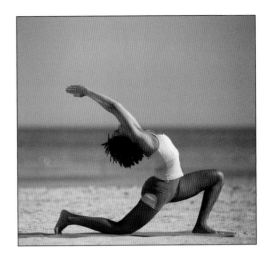

Yoga is a highly recommended activity to include in your cross-training, and will enhance your performance in all three TRI disciplines. Once considered an ancillary endeavor, yoga is now an important tool in the training arsenal for many professional triathletes due to both the physical and mental benefits. Yoga keeps muscles and tendons supple and improves flexibility, which is key for preventing injuries. Your core strength and balance develops significantly, while your mental focus is sharpened.

If you are already engaged in a workout program that you enjoy such as Crossfit© or a video training program like P90X© or T25©, don't hesitate to continue with it. If it is a daily program and you're cramped for time, you could reduce the program to every other day or even a couple times per week. Most programs such as these will give you many cross-training benefits. If you find yourself overly fatigued, back off. Listen to your body.

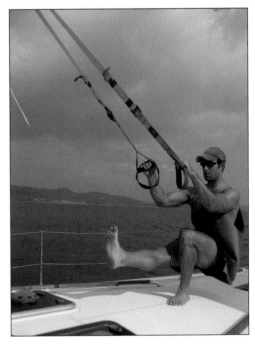

Beyond Fitness

TRI is more than just a way to become physically fit. When you become involved with triathlons, you'll notice many changes in your life beyond the changes in your body. Improved mental clarity, new relationships, and a more positive outlook on life are just a few of the benefits that you can look forward to once you make TRI part of your life.

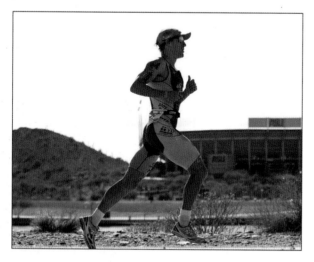

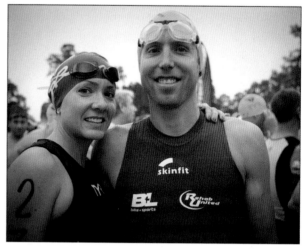

The TRI Mindset

We live in a busy world with many distractions. Some days feel full of chaos, packed with stress, worry, and grief. TRI teaches you to be present in the present. When you're training or racing, you must focus on the *now* of things:

> *How's my pace?*
>
> *How's my form?*
>
> *Don't step in that pothole.*
>
> *It's time to drink some water.*

When your attention is in the present, you feel stillness, calmness, and a sense of peace. The mind is a powerful thing. TRI can help you better understand the mind-body connection and help you relax.

New Faces, New Friends

Beyond balance and inner peace, TRI is full of social opportunities. You may have a different workout partner for each activity: pool swimming, open-water swimming, bike riding, trail running, yoga, and resistance training. You may meet with certain groups for certain workouts.

Spinning or other cycling classes are also great ways to be social. You might find an instructor you love or attend with some friends. These classes can be focused and intense, but there's also room for interaction and bonding.

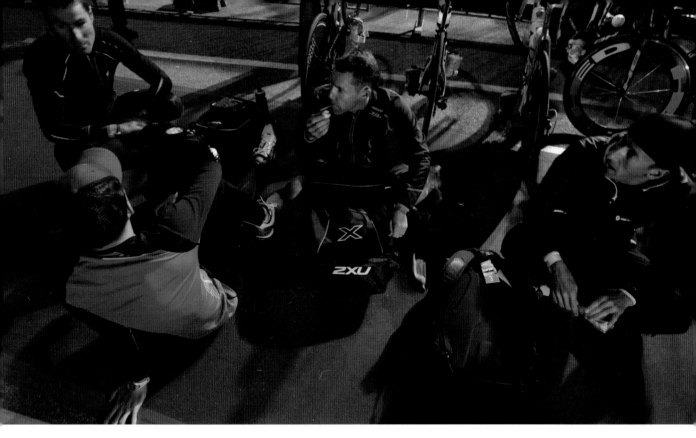

TRI Clubs

Many triathletes get involved with local TRI clubs. This is a great way to meet people, forge relationships, learn, and have fun. Clubs often have websites with useful information about races and group events. They typically get together weekly, monthly, or quarterly. Some hold mini-races followed by food, drink, and socializing. Other advantages can include club member discounts at various sport-related businesses.

Some clubs tread outside the normal TRI training modes and do things such as rock climbing, skiing, hiking, or anything members are interested in. It's great to mix things up, socialize, and let loose. The TRI community has its own subculture. They look like everyone else, but often possess many of the following characteristics:

- Confidence
- Adaptability
- Mental toughness
- Focus
- Emotional stability

Triathletes tend to have the "anything is possible" attitude.

Spirit and Emotion

Health is made up of five main components:

- Physical
- Mental
- Social
- Emotional
- Spiritual

When we are firing on all cylinders, we have the greatest level of life quality, happiness, and self-actualization. TRI has the potential to improve each of the five facets of health. We've already discussed some of the physical, mental, and social aspects, but how does TRI affect emotional and spiritual health?

An Emotional Experience

Training and competing in triathlons can tap into a wide range of emotions. The physical struggles can bring pain, fear, and doubt, while the accomplishments can bring overwhelming joy. Triathletes are often moved to tears when crossing the finish line during the most difficult races and triathlons. There's an incredible rush of genuine feeling that seems to come out of nowhere. Elation, sadness, relief, pride, and suffering all slam into you at once, and the tears start flowing.

TRI provides a vehicle to experience emotions on a new level. Some say the compulsion to compete in the sport stems from the power of the emotional charge one experiences during training and competing. Perhaps it is a trigger for the flow of endorphins. Emotion is a difficult thing to quantify and/or explain; it's best understood through your own experiences.

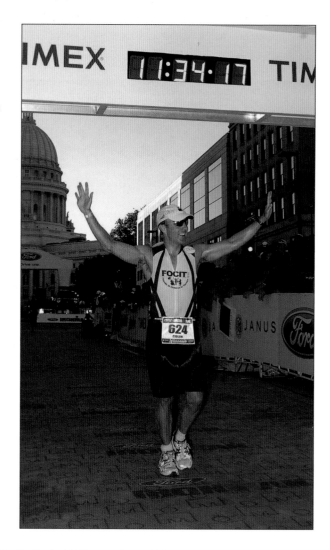

Facing Your Fears

One emotion you may feel in connection with TRI is fear. Fear shows up differently for everyone. Some may fear open water swims, fast descents on the bike, or more generally, their overall race results. In order to make the best of your TRI experience, you need to deal with any fears that may be lingering. You need to accept the fear, act on it, or put it in perspective.

Accept the fact that you are nervous or scared. Most triathletes, if they're honest, will admit to being nervous about some aspect in TRI training or racing. It's okay. Nervousness is natural, and as long as you learn to control and channel this emotion, it cannot hurt you.

If your fear is more intense and focused, you'll need to face it head-on. If swimming in open water makes you feel panicked, you'll need to get past it if you want to be a triathlete. The best way to get over such a fear is by swimming the open water, over and over again. Go for a swim with someone who can help you through this challenge. Wear a wetsuit and only go out a short distance. Do this until you're confident. Being comfortable in everything you do is critical in your overall TRI success.

Gaining perspective on a situation can also play a key role. Ask yourself what you're afraid of and why. Then apply a sense of reality to it. If you're scared of not meeting your own race expectations, try to put that fear into context. If you don't finish in the time you wanted (don't forget: we advocate not having a time goal) or if you're not feeling the way you wanted, then you'll have a tremendous learning opportunity. You may learn something about your training strategy and how you can adjust it the next time around. As long as you document any lessons learned and utilize them next time around, almost all race experiences can only help you. Putting perspective around the fear should help you control it. In the grand scheme of things, is this fear worthy of my time and stress? Is it a big deal? Perhaps once you take a step back, you'll realize the fear is superficial and you can get past it.

Tapping into the Spiritual

The spiritual component is closely related to emotion. When we are faced with adversity, struggle, and pain, we tend to look deep within for answers. We are looking for strength from our soul. It is in those times, the times we want to quit, when we push on through. It's the voice inside that cries *NEVER give up!* When we learn we can tap into this inner power, we grow, evolve, and discover a truer version of ourselves. This may happen during training or racing in any distance of TRI in which you really have to push yourself.

At one point or another, you will need to tap into this potential. Your body will find an extra level that you did not know was there. There will be times when you want more than anything to quit and go eat a cheeseburger; at those times you'll need to remember why you decided to start this journey.

Can I Do This?

There are no physical prerequisites for you to start in TRI. You don't have to be in good shape, or know how to swim, ride a bike, or run. You just have to be willing to exert some effort and learn. For most people, swimming is the most daunting, but if you commit yourself to learning, you will succeed. Take swim lessons at a local gym or health club. Once you've got the basic front crawl stroke down, you just need to practice and work on your endurance.

Biking and running are usually skills developed in early childhood. If you have graduated to adulthood without the ability to ride a bicycle, it's time to find a good friend who can help you learn. This will involve a lot of trial and error, and you will probably sustain some bumps and bruises, but if you're dedicated, you can do it.

Beyond the basic skills of swimming, biking, and running, only you know what you want to achieve. Would you like to train for a triathlon and not necessarily compete in one? Do you want to lose some weight and adopt a healthier lifestyle? Do you feel inspired to complete an Olympic-distance triathlon after watching the last summer Olympics?

This is one area where we cannot offer too much advice. Only you can match your personal goal to a race distance and training schedule. People who don't really want to commit to a scheduled race or who are just starting out in all three sports might want to look into a super sprint or sprint triathlon; an Olympic-distance race and training program might be a stretch.

If you've already done a few sprint triathlons and are comfortable with all three sports, consider an Olympic-distance triathlon or longer. Keep in mind that longer distances mean more time spent training, so try to figure out how much time you'll have available for training per week, and compare that with the hours associated with the different training programs outlined later in the book. Only you can decide what's best for you.

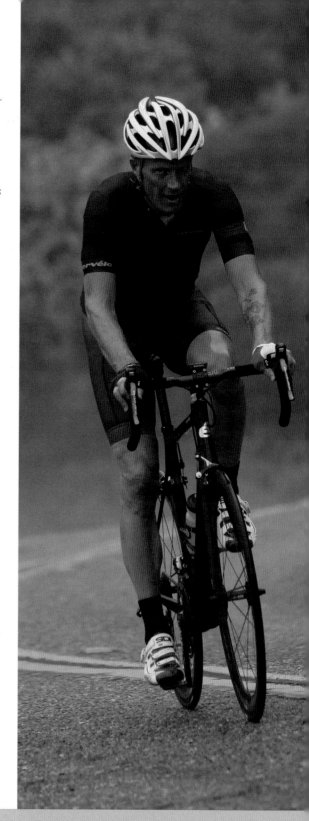

Setting Goals

Now that you've decided to take this journey, figure out exactly what your goals are. The most important element of setting goals is to make sure they are measurable. Distance and time make for easy goal tracking, as opposed to just saying you want to "get faster." Goals are meant to inspire and motivate you, so be realistic when setting them. You want to aspire to your goals without making them too overwhelming or daunting.

Your overall goal for a triathlon might be completion of a specific race or achievement of a specific time. However, setting smaller goals is important, too. Make weekly goals for your training such as, "I want to swim laps continuously for 15 minutes without stopping," or "I want to run a mile without taking a break." These "mini" goals will benefit you significantly within the bigger context of training and racing.

Once you figure out your goals, write them down and display them. Whether on your fridge, by your alarm clock, or posted on your desk at the office, this visual aid will help keep you motivated and remind you of what you've mentally declared. It's especially good on days when you're having trouble keeping to your workout schedule. Sometimes we need such a tool to give us a little nudge.

Goals for the week

◇ Train five days in each discipline.

◇ Take a yoga class.

◇ Swim three extra laps during my training sessions.

◇ Tackle a new hill on a course on the bike.

◇ Run three miles without stopping.

◇ Start each day with warm water with lemon.

Choosing Your Race

If this is your first TRI, you probably want to err on the side of caution and choose a race that might be a little shorter instead of going for one that might be too long. There's nothing worse than putting unnecessary pressure on yourself to compete in a race for which you don't have ample time to prepare. This doesn't mean you won't be able to take on one of the longer races soon, but you might want to complete a shorter race first to prepare for that longer one.

Another reason to start off with a shorter race is to build your confidence. If your end goal is a longer race, completing a shorter TRI helps you gain a sense of accomplishment and knowledge that you can finish. After that, your goal might be to improve your time or increase your race distance. After you successfully complete each one, you'll have that much more belief in yourself and your abilities to get to the next level.

Timing

One of the biggest considerations when deciding what race you want to shoot for is how long you have until race day. Will you have enough time to prepare for the distance you want to conquer? Will your schedule allow for some adjustments in the short term? Perhaps you have many months before your goal race. With proper planning, you can make any race happen with enough time ahead of you.

The longer the race you're preparing for, the more time you need to train. If your goal is to compete in a sprint triathlon, you'll be able to prepare in three months. If you want to go for the Ironman distance, you'll need about six months. These amounts of time can be adjusted based on your fitness level.

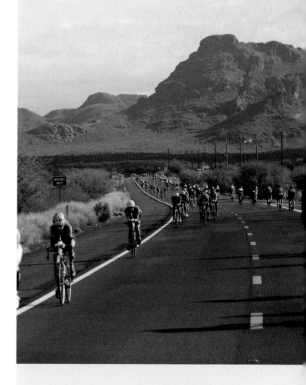

Average Weeks Needed to Prepare for Triathlon

Distance	Training Time
Super-sprint	4 to 10 weeks
Sprint	6 to 14 weeks
Olympic	8 to 16 weeks
Half-Ironman	10 to 20 weeks
Ironman	16 to 30 weeks

Location

Now that you have some idea about the distance and training time you need for the race you've set your sights on, you can decide where you want to do it. Most likely, you can find some races in your general area. However, they might not match your distance requirements. If you're looking to travel to your race, you'll have thousands of options around the planet.

Staying close to home has many advantages. You're able to organize and reorganize your equipment several times the night before the race, sleep in your own bed, use your own alarm clock to wake up in the morning, and prepare whatever breakfast you would like in your own kitchen.

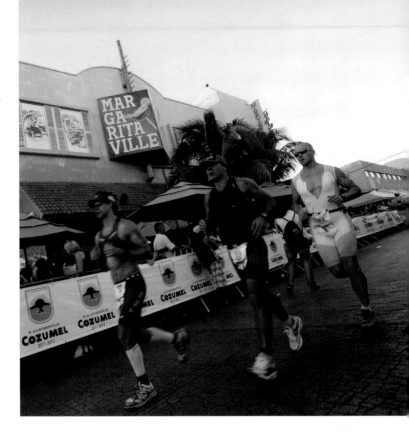

On the other hand, completing a triathlon in a faraway place can be a great way to get a special perspective on a travel destination. Going to another location can make you feel more "official." Experiencing a race in a different place might help your mind focus on the big day because you're removed from other distractions and concerns that might cause worry in your home environment. There's more cost and logistical planning associated with remote races, so you'll probably feel more invested and therefore more likely to follow through with your training and racing. Some extra considerations:

- Traveling can add stress
- Beyond clothing, you'll have to get your bike to the race venue (or use a rental)
- Your lodging and food choices might be out of the ordinary
- Distant venues may limit the participation of friends and family who would otherwise come to cheer you on

Whatever you choose to do, make sure to sign up and make any necessary reservations as early as possible. Do not procrastinate—races and hotels fill up. You don't want to miss out on your race plan because you were too slow on the draw.

Sprint-Distance Triathlon

Sprint-distance triathlons are a bit longer than super-sprints, but there is no clear distinction. Distances for each leg of a sprint triathlon vary, but usually fall within a certain range.

> Swim: 375 to 750 meters (0.23 miles to 0.47 miles)

> Bike: 10 to 22 kilometers (6.2 miles to 13.2 miles)

> Run: 3 to 5 kilometers (1.9 miles to 3.1 miles)

Who Should Compete?

The sprint triathlon is a great first race distance. A 750-meter swim course might be a challenge for a beginning swimmer, but with proper training it is doable. This distance is also good for those who have competed in the past and want to get back into the race groove, or those who are testing the recovery of an injury. The sprint is one of the most popular triathlon distances and can be found in most areas.

Transitions and Pacing

Because sprint distance triathlons are relatively short, taking a long time during transitions will add significantly to your finishing time. This shouldn't be a concern; just something to be aware of.

When the gun goes off in distance sprint race, the adrenaline can help carry you through the entire swim. This might cause you to push your body too hard while in the water. Be aware that this can happen, catch yourself, relax, and recover so your race won't be affected. If you pop out of the water, change, grab your bike, and start cranking away on the pedals, check yourself and slow down. Adrenaline is a great energy booster, but don't depend on it to carry you through the entire race. Relax and save some for the run. Learning your pace comes with experience.

Time to Complete and Recovery

A sprint triathlon can take anywhere from less than one hour to two hours or more, depending on your fitness level. It won't take up your entire day, and you should be able to recover relatively quickly with proper nutrition and hydration. The next day, you should feel minimal soreness.

Olympic-Distance Triathlon

Olympic-distance triathlons are exactly that: events the distance of the triathlon that takes place in the Olympics. Unlike the sprint-distance triathlon, the distances for each leg are standardized.

>Swim: 1.5 kilometers (0.9 miles)

>Bike: 40 kilometers (24 miles)

>Run: 10 kilometers (6.2 miles)

Who Should Compete?

The total distance of the Olympic-distance triathlon is over 50 kilometers (30 miles) long, so it is not ideal for a first timer. However, it could be a first race for those willing to put in the time it takes to prepare. This is also a great practice race for people who are training for a longer triathlon later in the season.

Transitions and Pacing

The swim portion of an Olympic-distance triathlon is too long to be fueled solely by adrenaline. This is a distance that will require proper pacing. If you keep up an unreasonable pace throughout the entire swim and the beginning of the bike, it will negatively impact you either during the second half of the bike segment or on the run.

Going out too hard happens to the best of us. The key to overcoming the tendency to push too hard is to be aware that it will happen and be prepared to reign yourself in when it does. When you realize you're going faster than you had planned, just take a moment to relax, slow down, and settle into your pace.

As with the sprint, your transition is not a time to relax. Practice transitions often so you can smoothly change the necessary gear and move onto the next sport.

Time to Complete and Recovery

This course could take you from under two hours to four hours or more to complete, depending on your pace. A race of this length requires a plan for taking in fluids and possibly fuel (we'll discuss nutrition on the move later in the book). You will definitely need a little more recovery time after this race than after shorter events, and your muscles will probably feel fatigued for the rest of the day. Be prepared for some soreness the next day as well.

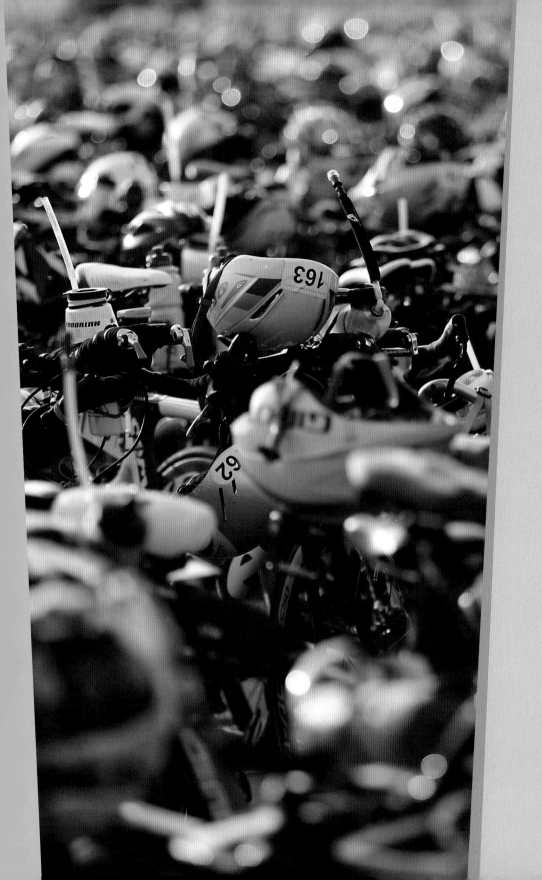

Equipment

You don't need too much stuff to participate in triathlon. A bike, helmet, swimsuit, goggles, and shoes are the bare necessities. However, there are seemingly endless options available, and it's possible to spend thousands of dollars on top-of-the-line items. How do you know what's essential and what's not?

The keys for selecting triathlon equipment are comfort and efficiency. You obviously want to be comfortable while you're training. If your shoes are too tight or your bike hurts your back when you ride it, you'll be less apt to continue with your training program.

Efficiency is also an important factor in equipment choices. Well-designed shoes and light-weight bikes can make your TRI experience easier and more enjoyable, but only you can decide how much each step up in efficiency is worth. This part will help you make equipment choices that maximize comfort and efficiency for your training program and lifestyle.

Swimsuits

Almost everyone has a swimsuit somewhere in his or her wardrobe. It need not be sleek or stylish. As your level of interest in triathlon increases, or if your environment demands it, you may want to upgrade to some better gear, but you really don't need much to start.

Your swimsuit can be loose or tight, big or small, one piece or two. However, while there are no hard and fast rules, most people who swim for fitness and training choose to wear a one-piece, form-fitting suit. This enables you to cut through the water more efficiently. A bulky suit increases drag as you slice through the water, which slows you down slightly. Although this additional drag probably won't make or break your swim time, it is something to keep in mind.

In the sport of swimming, streamlined suits are more or less expected for both men and women. If you are working with a swim coach, a tighter suit will allow your coach to see your form more easily as he or she critiques your overall technique. Helpful tips and small corrections in your form will definitely cause your time to improve both in the swim (you'll be moving faster) and in the rest of your triathlon (you'll have wasted less energy in the water).

When selecting a swimsuit, comfort is the most important factor. Don't buy the most expensive suit, or a certain brand just because your favorite triathlete wears it. It must work for you. Swimsuits should be snug, and feel a little tight when you purchase them. After several swim workouts and subsequent launderings, your suit will lose a little elasticity.

Sporting goods stores typically have a broad selection of suits to choose from, and the prices will be average. Specialty brand shops will be more expensive. Both options usually have knowledgeable staff to answer questions, but it is a good idea to do some preliminary research online to narrow down some brands that could work for you, and make a decision after trying them on. Once you find a suit or brand that works for you, then you can shop online.

Men's Short Suit

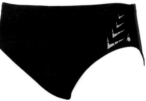

Men's Mid-Length Trunk

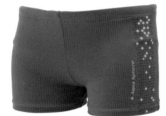

Men's Slim Trunk

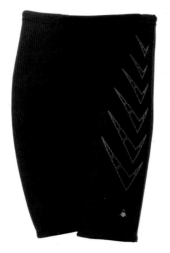

Women's Two-Piece Suit

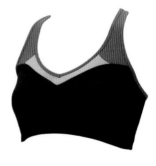

Women's Mid-Coverage Suit

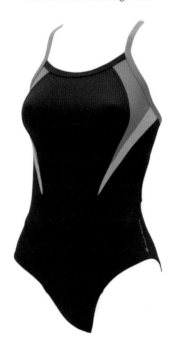

Women's Full-Coverage Suit

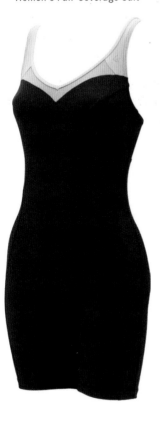

Swimsuits

Trisuits

Both men and women can wear trisuits, one-piece singlets that cover the entire body. Trisuits wick water away from your skin and bring it to the surface of the suit to get you dry as quickly as possible. These can be worn in warm water as a swimsuit and then stay on during both the bike and the run, eliminating the need to change clothes during transitions.

Although a trisuit is the epitome of efficiency, it might not be as comfortable as bike shorts while riding because the seat has less cushioning. If you're thinking about using a trisuit in a race, be sure you try it ahead of time to make sure that you're able to ride comfortably. One more thing to keep in mind: the single-piece construction of trisuits may make bathroom breaks more challenging.

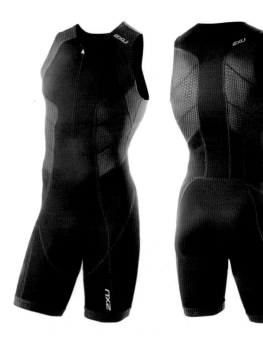

Men's Trisuit

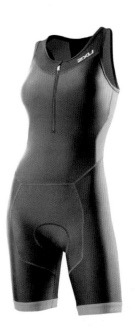

Women's Trisuit

Goggles

Beyond your swimsuit, goggles are the other necessity for swimming. Although they don't matter much while you're just messing around in the pool, if you're sharing a lap lane with another swimmer, doing flip turns during a workout, or in the middle of a pack of 50 swimmers at a triathlon, you need to be able to see what's going on around you.

A nice pair of goggles isn't very expensive and is a great investment that will make your experiences in the pool much better. Beyond keeping water (and chemicals) out of your eyes, you want the goggles to be comfortable and you don't want them to pinch in any spots.

Goggles come in a variety of shapes and sizes. Choose a pair that is comfortable for you.

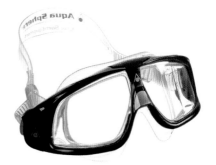 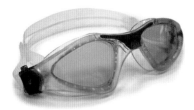 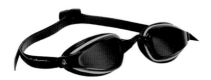

When purchasing goggles, it's worth seeking the advice of the employees at a specialty store. However, keep in mind that everyone's face is shaped differently. The perfect pair of goggles for one person might not even form a seal over another person's eyes. If you have the opportunity to try out a friend's goggles before you buy your own, go for it. If you get a pair and don't like it, buy another. Don't allow yourself to suffer through workouts with an inferior pair of goggles.

Many goggles are designed to resist fogging, but if you don't get that type, you can rub a little bit of saliva on the lenses to keep them fog-free. Keep a backup pair in your bag, just in case.

Wetsuits

If you'll be training or competing in cooler water, you'll most likely need a wetsuit. Even if the water temperature doesn't force you to wear a wetsuit, you might still want to consider it, as it will add buoyancy and efficiency.

Style

Triathletes, both male and female, generally use two main types of wetsuits:

Full wetsuits cover your core and extend down your arms to your wrists and down your legs to your ankles. They provide the most coverage, warmth, and buoyancy.

Sleeveless wetsuits are simply an armless full. Some prefer this option because shoulders and arms are less restricted.

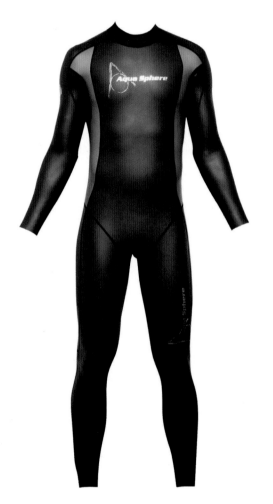

Men's Full Wetsuit

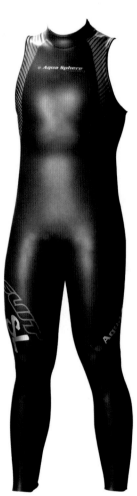

Men's Sleeveless Wetsuit

Short-sleeved wetsuits, and the short style wetsuits often used by surfers, are also available. If you already have this type of wetsuit, try it out while swimming and see what you think. No matter what type of suit you go with, keep in mind that warmth provided by a wetsuit is proportional to the amount of body coverage and the thickness of the suit.

The best type of wetsuit for you depends on how much warmth you want and how comfortable you feel in any of the options.

You can find wetsuits at most swimming or TRI stores, or you can order them online. Even if you plan to purchase online, find a store where you can try on a couple different options before ordering.

Fit

When you try on a wetsuit, it should feel tight. You don't want it to cut off circulation, but you don't want it to have "room to grow," either. Most people feel slightly uncomfortable when they first put one on, but you'll get used to it after a few swims. Some triathletes opt for the sleeveless version because it feels less constricting to them. It's all about your personal preference. There are several brands to choose from, but quality and comfort should be your main concerns. Pay special attention to the seams. You want a suit that won't unravel.

Lubrication

If you do purchase a wetsuit, lubrication becomes a necessity. The motions of swimming will cause your body to rub against the suit and could cause serious chaffing. Even the simple movement of turning your head to breathe while swimming in a wetsuit can cause irritation on the back of your neck after only a few minutes.

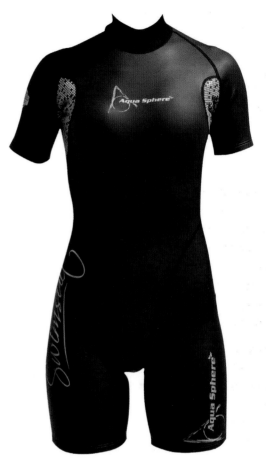

Women's Shorty Wetsuit

Swim Training Aids

Most people are accustomed to hopping in the pool, securing their goggles, and starting their swim workout. There is nothing wrong with that approach, and you would be able to prepare for your race that way. However, there are a few pieces of equipment that will allow you to go faster, hone your technique, or focus on specific parts of the body.

Buoys and Kickboards

For certain arms-only or legs-only swimming drills, you need a way to keep half of your body immobile (but afloat) as you swim across the pool. Pull buoys and kickboards do just that. You can squeeze a pull buoy between your thighs to keep your legs near the surface as you focus on specific upper body techniques. Kickboards keep your upper body afloat during leg drills.

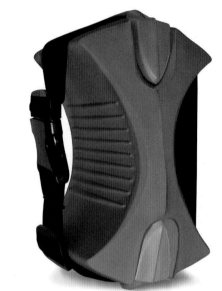

Pull Buoy

Although the pool where you decide to swim may already have these pieces of equipment for general use, some people prefer to bring their own. That way, they know they will always have access to one or both items when their schedule calls for it. If you bring your own, make sure you write your name on it with a permanent marker.

Several variations of these buoys and kickboards are available. Some look like futuristic, aerodynamic spaceships, and others just look like a piece of foam. The boring-looking pull buoy or kickboard does the exact same job, usually for a much lower cost. Don't be fooled by fancy looks and packaging when it comes to these swimming aids.

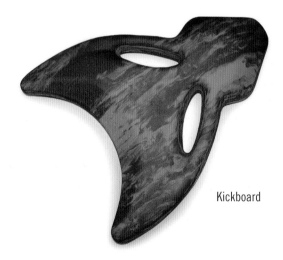

Kickboard

Hand Paddles and Fins

Hand paddles and fins might also be helpful in your training, but definitely are not necessary. These swim aids allow you to push against the water with a larger surface area, giving you more power to move forward. They increase your speed and make you feel the water sliding by you much faster. Neither of these is allowed in races, as it would give an unfair advantage, but both can be used to augment your training program.

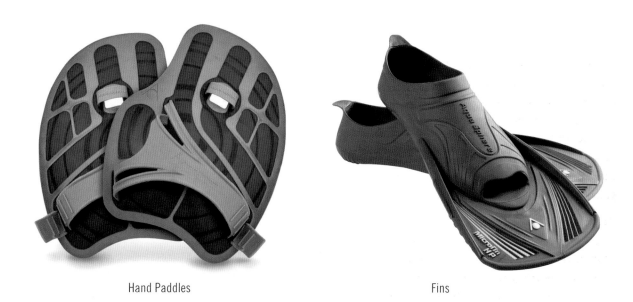

Hand Paddles   Fins

Special Pools

If money is no object, you may choose to investigate a never-ending pool, also called a swim spa or aqua trainer. These are smallish bodies of water with a constant current you can swim against. Similar to a treadmill, the speed of the current can be adjusted. Your goal is to stay stationary in relation to the pool boundaries. These pools give you a private, accessible, comfortable place to train for swimming, but they cost several thousand dollars and require regular upkeep and electricity. You should definitely be confident that swimming is something you'll be keeping up for years to come before you make this investment.

If you already have a pool, you can purchase a mountable device called a current generator, which creates a constant current similar to the never-ending pool. These devices are available for most types of pools.

Bike Types

With the variety of bike options available, choosing the right one for your triathlon may seem overwhelming. It doesn't have to be. If you already have a multi-speed bike, that might do just fine. Don't go out and spend a ton of money on a top-of-the-line bike right away. Get a tune up for your old bike and see how training goes.

If you're in the market for a new bike, we recommend one with several speeds. Beyond that, the bike you choose will depend on personal preference, along with the terrain on which you'll be riding and the types of races you plan to enter.

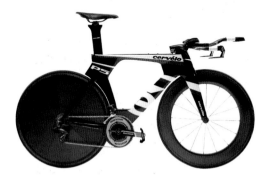

Triathlon (TRI) Bike

TRI bikes are designed to maximize speed and performance in a triathlon. With ideal geometry, a TRI bike will allow you to use your hamstrings more while cycling, which saves your quads for the run.

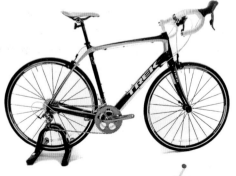

Road or Racing Bike

Road (or racing) bikes are also designed for speed, with narrow tires and drop-style handlebars. Road bikes are a good option for most triathlons, and you may find them more comfortable than a TRI bike.

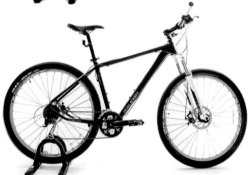

Mountain Bike

Mountain bikes have wide, knobby tires designed for dirt trails. These bikes are bulkier and heavier than road or TRI bikes, but if your race is a short one, they can suffice. Mountain bikes are also good for events with off-road terrain.

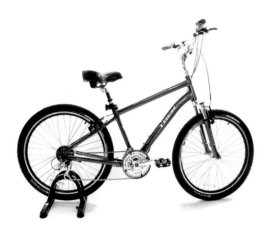

Hybrid Bike

Hybrid bikes are less bulky than mountain bikes, but still heavier and less efficient than a TRI or road bike. Hybrids can be used for shorter races or off-road races.

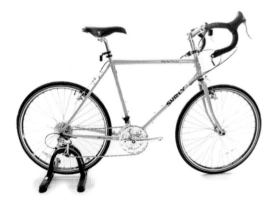

Touring Bike

Touring bikes are designed for stability and durability; not speed. You could use a touring bike for a shorter race, but it will be heavier and less ideal than other options.

Bike Material

Bike frames are constructed from several types of materials. The best material for your bike depends on several factors: your style of riding, your weight, and your terrain.

Aluminum is a widely used material. It is light, strong, and stiff, three important qualities. It is also less expensive than some other materials.

Carbon steel is another commonly used bike material. It is a strong and long-lasting option. However, it is heavier than most other materials.

Chromoly steel is a light and strong steel material. It is considered a responsive material and offers flex while maintaining form.

Titanium is lighter than steel and just as strong. It has significant ability to flex and maintain its shape. It is generally a more expensive option.

Carbon fiber is currently the most sought after and prestigious of all bike materials. It is the lightest of the options, tough, and pliable. While it has impressive responsive "give," which acts like shocks on rough roads, carbon fiber is also less resilient compared to the other materials. Carbon fiber bikes are typically higher priced.

It comes down to what resonates with you, what's comfortable, and what price range is most reasonable for your lifestyle and involvement with triathlons.

Getting the right fit is as important to your performance as style and material. Consider a consultation with a bike-fitting specialist when purchasing a bike.

Specialized Wheels and Aerobars

Unless you're an elite athlete, you don't need to worry too much about improving your aerodynamics for a shorter race. However, if you're registered for a longer race, you may want to consider a few upgrades for your handlebars and wheels that will increase efficiency and add comfort during long training rides and races.

Race Wheels

While unnecessary for the beginner in a shorter race, race wheels are something to consider if you want to improve your speed. Thick-rimmed (or deep-dish), three or four-spoke, and disc wheels are the main options. These wheels can be very expensive and are primarily used for racing rather than training. They are lighter than the standard spoke wheels and a bit more aerodynamic.

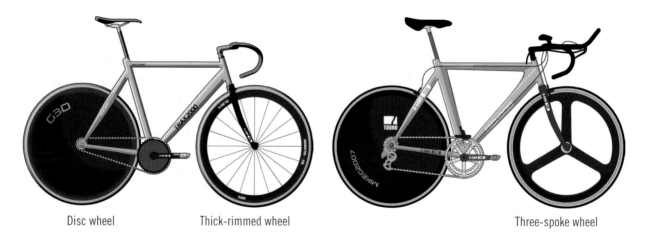

Disc wheel   Thick-rimmed wheel   Three-spoke wheel

Two types of tires can be used with most of these wheels: the standard tire (clincher) with an inner tube, or a tubular tire. The tubular tire is a single piece that's wrapped around the wheel frame and inflated (not a tube/tire combo). Special wheel glue is used to adhere the tire to the wheel. These tubular tires are much more expensive than the standard replacement tube for a clincher tire. However, after you get used to them, tubular flats can be changed more quickly.

While disc wheels offer great aerodynamic benefits when you're riding into the wind and for longer distances, if a strong side wind blows, things can get precarious. Under some extreme wind conditions, race directors will ban disc wheels before the start of the race. If you plan to use disc wheels, have a backup plan in place.

Aerobars

Aerodynamic handlebars, or aerobars, are a great addition for any cyclist who will be riding long stretches on relatively flat terrain. They can improve both comfort and efficiency.

Aerobars have only been around since 1989. They offer the rider a way of "cheating the wind" with a combination of handlebars and elbow supports that position the head and shoulders lower and more forward than regular handlebars. Ideally, your elbows will be close to a right angle, and most of the weight from your head and shoulders will transfer straight through your upper arms into the elbow supports. The lower your upper body, the more aerodynamic you become. Although you may not notice a change on a short ride on a windless day, the benefits will be very evident on a long ride or anytime the wind is in your face.

There are different options when it comes to aerobars. Regardless of the manufacturer or the style, the goal is to get you down into that aerodynamic position. One type of aerobars called "extensions" can be bolted onto the top, center area of your current handlebars. Integrated aerobars actually replace the old handlebar setup on your bike and leave you only with aerobars (no "drop" section on the handlebar). Many TRI bikes are sold with this second type of aerobar. If you're not sure you want to go the aero route, start with standard handlebars; you can always buy extensions later.

Both types of aerobars come in various sizes. You'll need to get sized properly before you purchase. The right size is based on the length of your forearm. Here's how to determine the right size:

1. Place your elbow on a flat surface and point your forearm up toward the ceiling.

2. Make a fist and then measure the distance from where your elbow rests on the flat surface to your highest knuckle.

3. Take that measurement to your local bike shop or compare with an online chart.

If you are new to triathlons, aerobars may not be worth the investment. They're also not recommended if you live in a very hilly area that will prevent you from relaxing in the aero position. In these cases, you can stick with the standard handlebar setup.

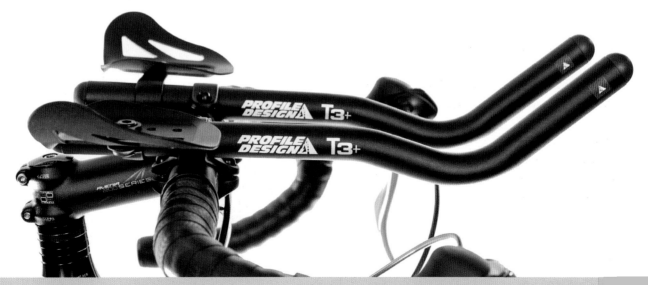

Specialized Wheels and Aerobars

Helmets

A helmet is not a discussion point. Get one. Get it before you go out for any riding. Helmets are not only for kids with overprotective parents. You are no longer riding around the block on the sidewalk; you're becoming a triathlete. You'll be out on the street with traffic around you, and you'll be going at speeds you may not have reached on a bike before. A helmet could save your life in an accident.

Get a helmet that you like and that fits comfortably. If you feel good wearing the helmet, you'll get into the habit more easily when you start off. Hopefully, you'll never have a fall, but if you ride long enough, you probably will. A helmet will do its best to protect your head so you can get up and ride another day.

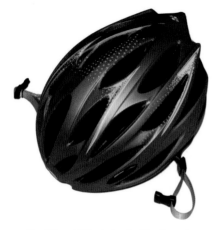

Traditional bike helmet with air vents

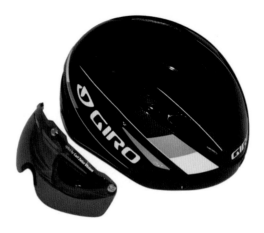

A more aerodynamic helmet with optional clip-on visor

Most bike helmets are not multi-impact helmets; they need to be replaced after one serious impact. It's a good idea to replace a helmet that's hit the ground or been in a small crash, because deficiencies in the helmet may exist without being visible. Whatever helmet you choose to use, be sure it's certified by the U.S. Consumer Product Safety Commission (CPSC). Check the label or box for this certification.

Glasses

You shouldn't ride without sunglasses. Beyond blocking the sun's harmful rays, they also keep your eyes safe in other ways. Even an average rider can easily get up to 30 miles per hour (48 kilometers per hour) going down a long hill. Your eyes must be protected when you're going at that speed. Besides just wind, passing car tires could send small pebbles flying or an insect could find its way into your eye. Be sure the glasses you select fully cover your eyes (wrap-around) and block UV rays.

Generally, polarized lenses are recommended. These lenses will protect your eyes from UV rays, and also eliminate the glare you'll encounter in bright light. Consider what lens color is best for your needs:

- Gray softens all colors but eliminates none.

- Yellow sharpens vision on cloudy or rainy days.

- Amber or brown are good in general, like gray.

- Clear are best for night riding.

- Darker lenses are good for bright light.

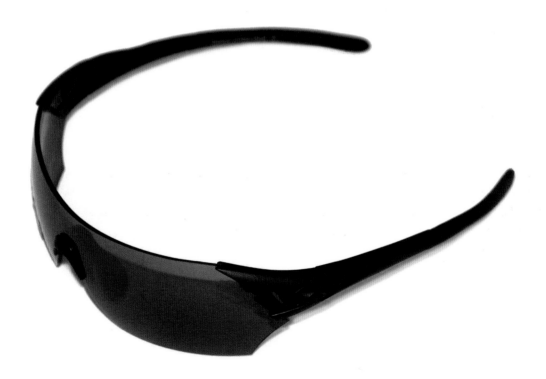

Pedals and Shoes

If you're going to make any upgrades to your bike, the pedals are a good place to do it. The flat pedals that come standard with most bikes only allow you to generate power on the down stroke. To truly be efficient, you want to be able to move your feet in a circle, instead of just pushing down every pedal revolution. You can achieve this efficiency in a few different ways.

Pedal Straps or Toe Clips

Pedal straps or toe clips are relatively cheap and add a great deal of efficiency to your pedal strokes. The straps or clips attach to your existing pedals and your foot slides into the area created by a clip over your toe, or the arch created by a strap over the front of your foot. Because they hold your foot in place, clips or straps allow you to transfer power from your legs to the pedals in three directions: you can push down, push forward, and pull up with your legs as the pedals rotate around the crank. You don't need special shoes to use toe clips or pedal straps.

Clipless Pedals and Bike Shoes

For greater pedaling efficiency, you can use clipless (also called clip-in) pedals and bike shoes. With a clipless system, cleats are fitted to the soles of special cycling shoes, which then snap onto the pedal, securing the shoe in place (like a ski boot in its binding). With your foot securely fastened to the pedal, you're able to move your foot in a truly circular motion and use every possible directional muscle in your leg to power your ride. Plus, you won't have to worry about your foot slipping out of a strap.

The process of clipping in is usually achieved by pressing firmly down on the pedal. To release your foot, you usually twist your heel out and back. However, there are several different styles of clipless pedal systems and they all have slightly different mechanisms. If you can, test a few to see which one feels most comfortable.

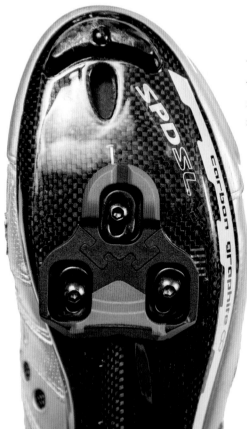

The cleat attaches to the bottom of specially designed shoes.

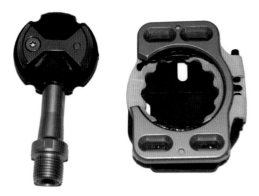

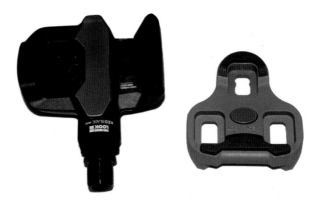

Speedplay is one brand of clipless pedals and cleats. There are other options available that range in price, material, and weight.

SPD is another popular type of pedals and cleats.

Riding with Toe Clips and Clipless Pedals

Some people are nervous about having their feet attached to the bike and are afraid they'll fall over the first time they try to stop. This may happen. If you decide to get toe clips or clipless pedals, practice starting and stopping several times in an empty parking lot or other flat spot without any traffic before setting out on the road.

Even after several practices, you may one day forget to unclip when coming to a stop. If you fall over while out in public, don't panic! It has happened to almost everyone at some point or another. Your first reaction will probably be to try to get up right away, but your feet might still be attached to the bike. Stay calm, but quickly unclip or slide your feet out of the straps. Then ease out from under the bike, stand up, right yourself, and quickly get out of the road. Then, when you're out of harm's way, check for any injuries. If only your pride is hurt, let go of any embarrassment and get moving again.

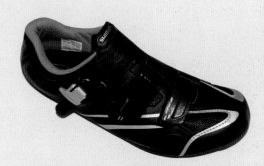

These cycling shoes have both Velcro straps and a ratcheting adjustment buckle.

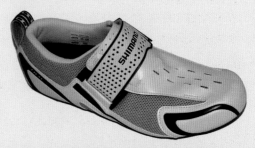

Shoes with only a Velcro strap can be slightly faster to get on and off.

Hydration and Storage Equipment

Bottle Cage

Depending on the distance of your ride, you'll probably want to have some sort of water bottle holder (cage) on your bike. Most people need to drink at least one 24-ounce (710 mL) bottle of liquid during an hour of biking. If don't plan to bike that long, you might be able to get away without a water bottle cage. However, you can get one for only a few dollars, so we highly recommend you add at least one to your "needs" list.

You can mount cages in a couple different ways. Most bikes already have pre-drilled holes inside the frame where a cage can be added. Another option is to get an additional attachment that allows mounting behind your saddle. If you're going to be out for long rides where you'll need several bottles, you might need both.

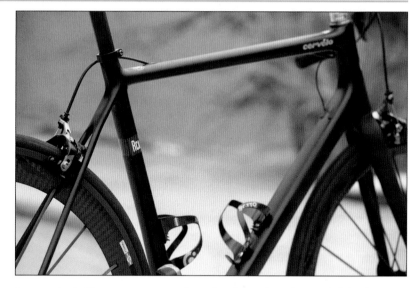

Frame water bottle cages are commonly used and come in various materials, shapes, and prices.

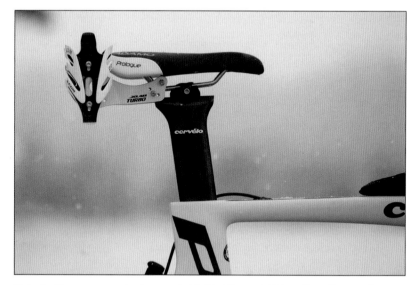

Water bottle cages can also be mounted behind the seat. This option offers greater aerodynamic efficiency.

Hydration Systems

Fancy water bottles or hydration systems are also nice to have, but are by no means necessary. Some water bottles fit right between your handlebars and enable you to drink straight out of a straw while in the aero position. A full bottle on the front of your bike could affect your steering, so if you decide to go this route, be sure to practice your turns before riding in a crowd. Other water systems carry the water behind and under the seat and have a longer hose that reaches up to your mouth. The choice depends on your goals and your preferences. If you're going to be in the aero position most of the time, you might want a straw-based system. For shorter races, or if you're doing a lot of climbing, a frame-mounted bottle cage might be best.

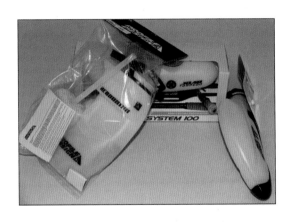

Seat Packs and Frame Bags

Seat packs and frame bags are great for carrying small pieces of equipment or food while out on a ride. A seat pack attaches below and behind the seat and usually has room for a spare tube, a bike tool, and some spare cash. It is also a great spot to stash your cell phone if you don't want to carry it in a pocket or smartphone holder (put it in a sealable plastic bag to protect it from weather and sweat).

A frame bag typically sits on your top bike tube, just behind the handlebars and is secured by Velcro straps. These bags are a great place to carry energy gels, bars, smartphone, or wallet. Neither of these items should cost very much, and both offer loads of convenience.

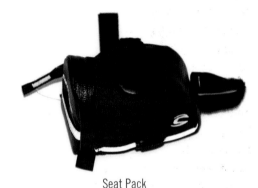

Seat Pack

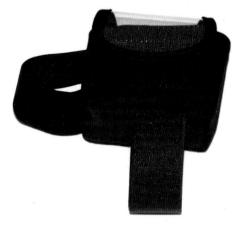

Frame Bag

Bike Apparel and Other Equipment

Shorts

Bike shorts make long rides on small seats much more comfortable. These shorts are made of a body-hugging material that not only reduces wind resistance, but also wicks away sweat. Many types have bands of silicone or other material along the inner edge of the leg opening that prevents the shorts from rolling or slipping as you ride. The most important thing, however, is that bike shorts have a pad called a chamois (pronounced "shammy") that cushions your bottom. The cut and padding of the chamois is gender specific for best fit. The shorts might feel a bit uncomfortable at first, but trust us: everyone is wearing them.

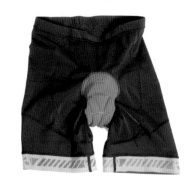

Jersey

When most people first get bike shorts, they elect to get a matching jersey, too. Jerseys are available in short-sleeve, long-sleeve, and sleeveless versions; fit close to the body to improve aerodynamics; and assist in wicking away sweat. They also have the added bonus of one to three pockets in the back or on the sides. These pockets are very handy when you need to carry snacks, cell phones, or anything else out on a ride.

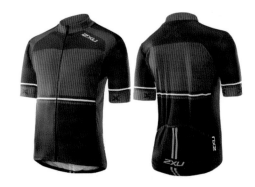

Gloves

Bike gloves are another option. They have some padding around the palms to cushion your hands and cutoff fingers to maintain dexterity. Some triathletes feel gloves add a level of comfort, but others don't use them at all. It's all a matter of personal preference.

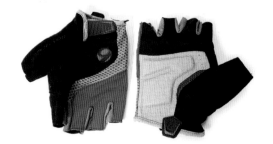

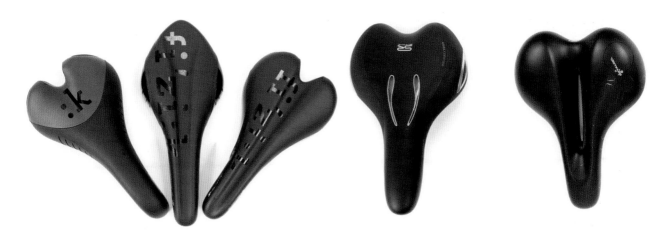

Saddle

A standard bike saddle, or seat, might not look or feel comfortable at first, but it's designed to allow for proper form and you'll get used to it over time. There are many different choices on the market that vary in material, shape, and price. For example, some have an anatomic central opening that can help alleviate some pressure. Experiment with different types to find what works best for you; it's an individual preference.

Indoor Trainer

While it's ideal to do most of your biking outside, an indoor bike trainer can be very helpful when the great outdoors is too cold, hot, wet, or dark. They can also be used for specific workouts in a controlled environment. These devices elevate the back wheel of your bike and apply resistance to the tire, effectively turning your regular bike into a stationary bike. You can then ride and ride and get a great workout, without going anywhere. The resistance may be applied by a fan, magnet, or fluid. Fan indoor trainers are at the lower end of the price range but can get very loud. Magnet trainers are much quieter and not much more expensive than fan versions. The most expensive type of trainer, with fluid resistance, produces less heat buildup on your tires (and, therefore, less wear).

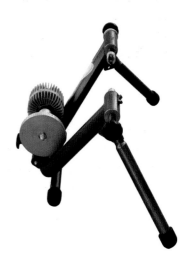

CO₂ Cartridges

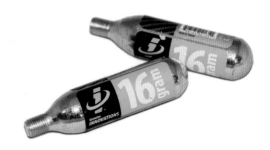

CO₂ cartridges and a regulator valve are two things that can make changing a flat a little less painful. The CO₂ cartridge is a cylinder, only a few inches long, that attaches to the small regulator valve. You put the other end of the valve device on your tire valve, creating a high-speed pump. Of course, you still need to replace the tube or tire as you normally would, but instead of having to pump up the new one manually, you simply use the compressed CO₂ to inflate the tire almost instantaneously. These things can be helpful anytime you have a flat, but you'll appreciate them the most during a race when time is of the essence.

Anytime you use CO₂ to inflate on a ride, be sure to check your tire pressure again when you get home. You might need to add a bit more air to hit the recommended pressure. Also, be aware that a CO₂ cartridge is usually only good for one full tire inflation.

Smartphone Apps and Bike Computers

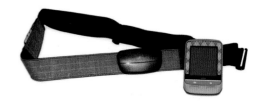

When you're out on a ride, it's helpful to have a way of tracking your distance, speed, and the number of rotations your pedals make per minute (RPMs). You can gather this data using a smartphone app or bike computer.

Smartphone apps often work in conjunction with sensors that you buy separately and attach to your bike. If you use your smartphone to track your stats, it's a good idea to purchase a waterproof case to mount to your handlebars.

If you don't have a smartphone, or don't want to use it while riding, you can get a relatively inexpensive bike computer. The most basic computers keep track of speed, distance, and time. More expensive options will also show your RPMs.

Knowing your RPMs helps you stay in the right training zones and keeps things efficient. This real-time readout can be very valuable. Whether you decide to get a computer or go the smartphone route, we recommend you try to utilize RPMs during your training.

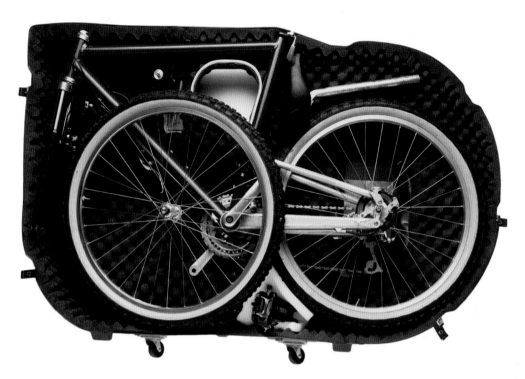

Bike Box

If you're going to be traveling on a plane to a race (or any plane trip where you want to bring your bike), a bike box is a necessity. The idea of a bike box is simple: to protect your bike as it's being tossed around by baggage handlers and conveyer belts. By disassembling some of the parts of the bike and securing them in a hard case, your bike's chances for survival increase drastically. If packed carefully with soft materials (like towels or bubble wrap), even the cardboard box the bike was originally packed in could suffice as a means of transport. Of course, that box might make it for only one trip, and it won't have wheels on the bottom to help you move it along smoothly.

More appropriate and convenient, although more expensive than a cardboard box, are hard case bike boxes. Some have separate wheel compartments, while others have one compartment for storing every piece of your bike. At a minimum, there's usually a way to lock down the bike frame. You can then position the wheels between the frame and the edges of the box. For extra padding, you can wrap different pieces of equipment with your old workout clothes. If you have extra space, you can carry other gear like energy bars or water bottles in the box, too.

Bike Rack

If you're traveling by car to a training location or a race, a vehicle mounted bike racking system might be in order. Many bikes have quick-release wheels and can fit into many trunks, but if you don't want to mess with the wheel, get a bike rack. They're relatively cheap, and enable you to pop your bike on and off quickly and easily. Remember to secure your bike both with bungee cords and some sort of locking device.

Running Shoes

Of the three triathlon disciplines, running requires the least amount of equipment. You. Shoes. Road. That's about it. When you were a kid, you probably ran with whatever shoes you had on that day, without a single thought about cushioning, stability, or durability. Now it is time to take those things into consideration.

To run, you need running shoes. These don't have to break the bank. Your local department store might have specials on great running shoes occasionally, but if you are brand new to running, you should consider going to a specialty running store for your first pair of shoes. A specialty running store employee will be able to evaluate both your foot type and running style and recommend a shoe that will compensate for any small issues and work with your foot shape and mechanics.

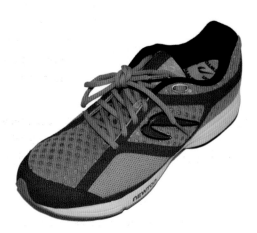

This running shoe has traditional tie laces.

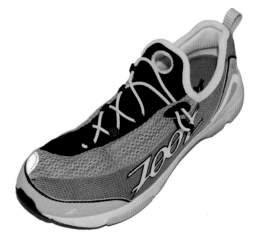

This shoe has tongue and heel pulls as well as a cinching lace system to save time during transition.

Some people swear by running shoeless, or with "barefoot" style shoes. The jury is still out as to whether this running philosophy is physiologically sound. If you choose to try this out, be sure to find a running store where an employee personally uses this style of shoe and can explain the risks and benefits to you.

The Best Shoe for You

When you are evaluated for a proper shoe, an expert will tell you that you are either a *pronator,* a *supinator,* or a *neutral* roller. These words are used to refer to the way the foot rolls when the ball of your foot strikes the ground as you run.

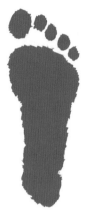

Pronation occurs if your foot strikes the ground, rolls inward and forward, and then pushes off the ball of your foot and big toe.

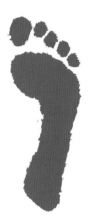

A **neutral** roll occurs when you strike and then roll through the middle of your foot and off the middle/front section of your foot.

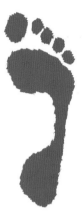

Supination occurs if your foot strikes the ground, rolls outward toward the outside of the foot, and then off the front-middle area of your foot and toes.

Runners with severe over-pronation or over-supination probably won't be able to compensate with just a shoe. These athletes might experience ankle or knee pain. If this happens to you, it is time to visit the foot doctor for corrective orthotics. All serious triathletes/runners either have orthotics or have been evaluated and told they do not need them.

In addition to the biomechanics of your foot strike and push off, you should also take the shape of your foot into consideration (what type of arch do you have, how wide is your foot, etc.). The least important aspect of your running shoes is appearance. Don't buy a shoe because you like how they look, or avoid a pair that's recommended because you hate the color.

Finding the Right Fit

At the most basic level, be sure any shoe you choose is snug but not tight. You should have about a thumb's width of "room to grow" from your toe to the end of the shoe. You want to be able to wiggle your toes a bit, and definitely don't want the end of your big toe rubbing against the tip of the shoe. The back of your foot should feel secure in the shoe as well. When you walk around, you don't want your heel lifting away from the shoe. A shoe like this won't give you adequate support and will probably cause serious blisters on the back of your ankle.

Your feet can swell up from your day's activities, so it's a good idea to shop for your shoes at the end of the day, when your feet are at their largest.

Running Apparel

There's a huge selection of running apparel out there. The key is to find clothing that fits well, feels comfortable, and is designed for athletic activity.

Shorts and Tights

Running shorts are a great addition to any runner's wardrobe. They are extremely light, come with a built-in liner, and often have a small inner pocket large enough to hold a key, an energy gel, or emergency cash. For cooler weather or for those who prefer a more close-fitting garment, running tights are another option. They're available in a variety of lengths and, like shorts, often have a small pocket on the waistband. As with most fitness apparel, both shorts and tights will wick sweat away from your body.

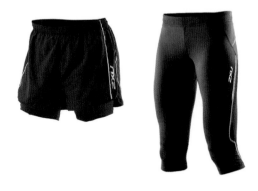

Tops

A running top made from a moisture-wicking material will be much more comfortable than cotton if you're planning to run more than a couple miles. Running tops are available in sleeveless, short-sleeve, and long-sleeve styles.

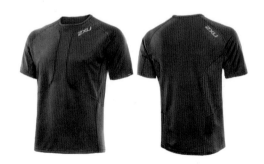

Hats

Hats are often overlooked by runners, but a running hat can really make your runs more comfortable. Look for a hat made specifically for running, with a sweatband-like lining that will keep the sweat out of your eyes. Most running hats are light colored on top to reflect sunlight and dark colored on the underside of the brim to absorb it.

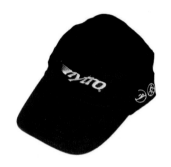

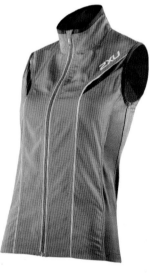

Cold-Weather Gear

Extra gear will be necessary if you're planning to run in the cold. Arm warmers, vests, tights, and jackets all help keep you warm on those cold days. Remember to protect your ears and hands with hats or ear warmers and gloves.

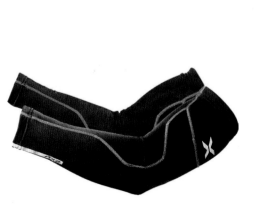

Lace Locks

Many triathletes use lace locks, spring-loaded gadgets that hold your laces in place, eliminating the need to tie your shoes.

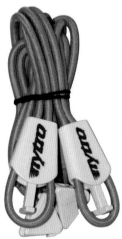

Sports Bra

A good sports bra is essential for women who run. Not only does it provide support, but it helps prevent breast pain and possible back strain. As with other running apparel, material, fit, and comfort are key.

Socks

Unless you already go sockless when running, you'll need some socks. It's worth paying a little more to get the thin, breathable, wicking type of athletic sock. Stay away from cotton, as it can cause blisters.

Fuel Accessories and Other Equipment

Nutrition Belts

You may want to consider a nutrition belt, or fuel belt, for longer runs. Most fuel belts hold multiple small plastic bottles. The bottles, which can be filled with energy gel or concentrated energy drink, are placed in holsters on the belt, and sit on the hips during the run. A fuel belt can be beneficial when run workouts last longer than an hour and you don't want to carry your nutrition in your hand or a pocket. If you're doing an Olympic-distance race or shorter, you'll be just fine without it.

A nutrition belt has space for fuel storage as well as compartments for personal items.

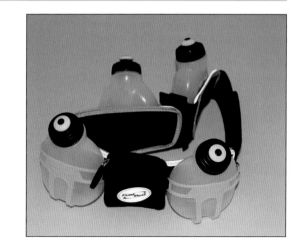

Hydration Systems

You might also decide to invest in a strap-on hydration system, either a bladder or belt style. The bladder option consists of a bag you can strap around your waist or wear on your back. The bag contains a bladder for hydration fluid, with a hose that can reach to your mouth. It's nice to always have fluids available, but the spot where the bag rests on your body will heat up. Be sure to add a lot of ice to the bladder on a hot day. The belt option usually straps around your waist and has a water bottle "holster." Both options are great to keep you hydrated out on long runs.

A flask with hand strap may also have options for additional storage.

Beware of the chaffing risk with hydration systems and fuel belts. When those belts or bags are laden with liquid, they may bounce along as you move, no matter how tightly you secure them. Be sure to apply lubrication where the main weight of the hydration system rests on your body, and test it on a short run first.

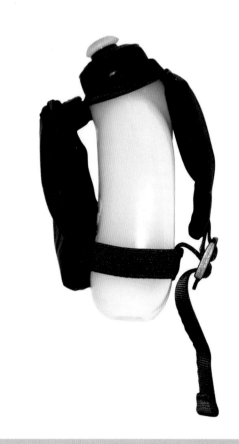

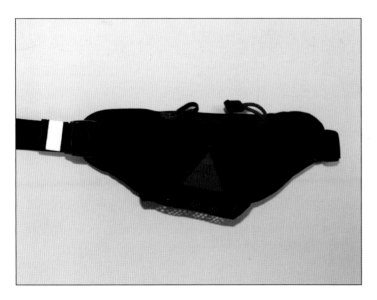

Running Belt

Running belts are another option for carrying small personal items. Although they are very small, many of them have expandable pockets, which allow you to even carry a cell phone. Gels, cash, salt tabs, and other small needs can also be stashed in the belt. Many of the belts on the market specifically claim that they will not chafe due to their design. If you go this route, try on a few before you buy.

GPS Watch

Although they will add some bulk to one of your wrists, many triathletes won't run without their GPS watch. Some of the more basic models will track your progress to give you data similar to what you'd get from your bike computer (avgerage speed, distance, calories burned, etc.). The more expensive, and usually larger, models will give you everything the basic watch offers, but include things such as a barometer and altimeter. One model even comes preloaded with skydiving software! The more expensive models will usually allow you to sync your workout (wirelessly or with a USB) to the web.

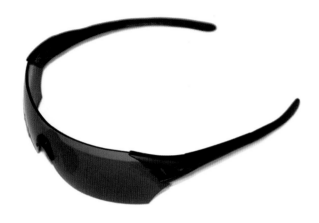

Sunglasses

Most people will use the same sunglasses for the run that they use on the bike. For running, you want your sunglasses to stay put. Most fitness style sunglasses will already have this attribute, but make sure to test out the bounce factor in the store before you buy.

Other TRI Equipment

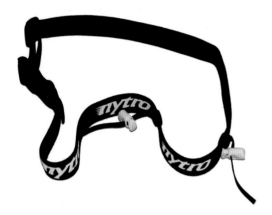

Race Belt

A race belt can be helpful in any race where you'll be wearing a race number (bib). These light, elastic belts clip around the waist and provide a place to pin your bib. Some triathletes prefer to use these instead of pinning the bib to their jersey because they can move the bib around their upper body by adjusting the belt. A race belt is also helpful if you plan to change your shirt during the race. Instead of having to unpin and re-pin your race bib, you can simply slide your race belt down to your hips as you change your shirt and you're ready to go.

Heart Rate Monitor

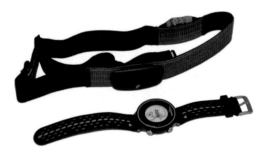

A heart rate monitor is a great addition to any triathlete's tool kit. Monitoring your pace and energy output via the heart rate is a reliable method for successful training. You'll first have to understand your heart rate zones, but self-testing for those is not too difficult. The monitor itself consists of a sensor and strap that wraps around your chest. It then sends a signal to a watch receiver you wear on your wrist. This simple monitor will tell you the time, date, and how fast your heart is working to keep you moving.

TRI Bag

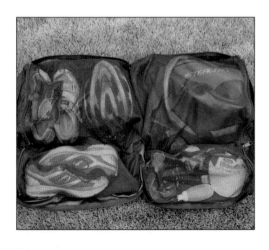

A TRI bag helps you get organized on your way to a race (or anytime you need to carry all your triathlon equipment with you). This backpack has specific compartments for shoes, helmet, wetsuit, etc. Mesh compartments on the outside of the bag can separate any wet gear from your other equipment. It has sections for everything, and can really help you organize your gear before leaving the house. A TRI bag enables you to easily tote all your gear on your back, which is handy if you have to park far away from the race venue or if you choose to ride your bike to a triathlon.

Sunscreen and Lubrication

When you compete in a triathlon, you'll already be pushing your body to the limit physically. You don't want to punish it further by neglecting to protect it from sun and chafing. Sunscreen and lubrication are two essential items for keeping yourself healthy and comfortable.

Sunscreen

Sunscreen is a must. Unless you plan to do all of your training and competing indoors, you should get a few good bottles of sunscreen. Be sure you get one that's water and sweat resistant and apply liberally before any outdoor activity. You might have to get a couple bottles per season to keep yourself protected.

If you're going to be training outdoors for more than an hour at a time, bring a sunscreen that is easily portable and reapply often. Remember that even "sweat-proof" sunscreen can come off during a hard workout, and be sure to cover the spots that will be exposed if your clothing shifts as you move (upper legs and arms, the back of your neck, and your ears).

Lubrication

When you compete in distance sports, you often sweat, and the repetitive movement of sweaty skin against skin, or skin against clothing, can cause painful chafing. Applying a specially formulated sports lubricant reduces friction and will keep you comfortable. The cost is minimal, and the pain it can save you is priceless. Spots where lube can protect you include:

- Underarms (while running or in a wetsuit)
- Back and side of the neck (while in a wetsuit)
- Inner thighs (while running or on the bike)
- Butt (where your cheeks touch the seat)
- Nipples (for men, while running)
- Spots where clothing is tight against the skin, such as a shorts waistband or bra straps (while running)

Sports lubricants are often packaged in sticks, like deodorant, which are very convenient to use. You can find these at almost any running, biking, or general sports store. One popular brand is Body Glide. If you're in a bind, you can also apply stick deodorant, petroleum jelly, or even cooking spray to reduce chafing.

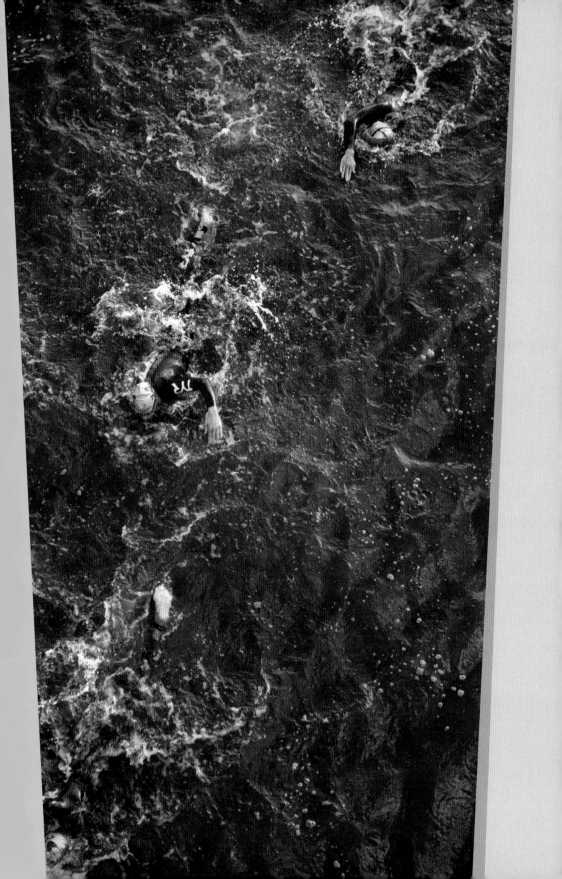

Swim

Although it is the first and shortest leg of the triathlon, swimming is often the most intimidating part of the race for beginners. This part will help allay your fears, and get you ready to be successful during the swim.

In the upcoming pages, you'll learn about the logistics of the swim portion of your race, as well as how to prepare for it, from the basics of breathing to very specific workouts.

Of the three triathlon sports, swimming has the least risk of possible overuse injuries. It's great for your cardio-respiratory systems (heart, lungs), your lower body (legs, hips, glutes), and upper body (core, arms, shoulders). The drills and workouts outlined in the upcoming sections will have you ready for your race in no time!

The Swim Stage

If you've never seen a triathlon, you probably have many questions about the actual logistics of the swim, which is the first leg of the race. How does it work?

Location

The swim portion of the triathlon most often takes place in open water. Along the coasts, most races start in the ocean. Inland, it may take place in a lake, river, or pond. In colder seasons or when smaller groups are putting on triathlons, the swim leg might take place at a local pool.

In an open water swim, nature will do as it pleases. You'll need to train in this type of environment so that you're prepared come race day. There may be a bit of a current and there might be some bigger waves. Keep in mind that everyone is dealing with the same conditions.

At the Start

There are two main types of starts: beach start and a water start. If your TRI is a beach start, you'll be all geared up, standing on the beach at the ready. When the gun goes off, everyone will sprint for the water. Use caution here. Don't risk diving into the water right behind another swimmer and getting kicked in the face.

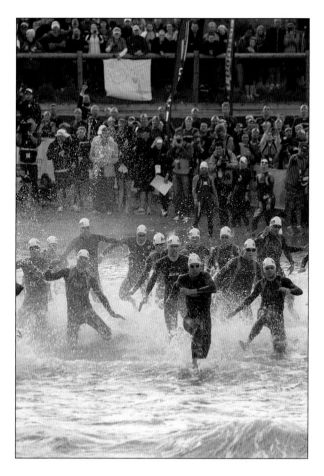

If your race is a water start, the official starting line will be at some point out into the water. Everyone will enter the water and wait anxiously for the gun. Usually the water will be shallow enough to stand, but in some races, you might need to tread water if you want to get close to the actual starting line. Again, if this idea causes undue stress, wait where you can still touch the bottom, and start swimming after the gun. You will not lose out on much time.

For either type of start, you will want to position yourself in the group based on your swimming experience and ability. Strong swimmers move near the front, average swimmers are in the middle, and less experienced swimmers are toward the back.

Staying on Course

Most beginners find that they do not swim in a perfectly straight line. To check yourself, close your eyes while swimming laps by yourself in the pool. Most beginners will veer slightly to one side.

In the pool, you have the black line painted along the bottom to keep you on course. When you're out in open water, you'll need to lift your head out of the water and look forward (instead of to the side) occasionally to "sight" your surroundings. Look for buoys, lifeguard towers, or any sort of landmark to check your position while you're on the move.

Some people decide to just follow the feet in front of them. If that is the route you take, you should still sight every once in a while to be sure you're not being led astray.

Bilateral breathing (taking breaths on both sides) also helps keep you moving in a straighter line. If you only breathe to one side you'll have a greater tendency to curve.

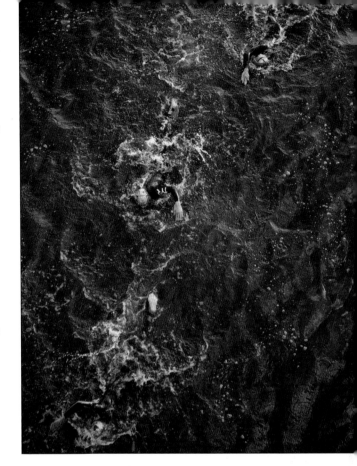

Course Layout

If your triathlon takes place in a pool, your course may be as basic as swimming in a lap lane for an allotted time. You might also have to swim a serpentine style course around the pool.

In open water swims, your course may be a simple out and back (turn around after rounding a buoy), or you might have to circle around a couple buoys before heading back to shore. In some of the longer races, you may have to do two laps around the course before coming in. Whatever the case, familiarize yourself with the course map ahead of time to avoid confusion while you're in the water.

Exiting the Water

As you are coming in from the swim, you'll be excited. After being horizontal for a while, it will feel strange to stand up and start running toward your transition to the bike segment (T1). You will hit either the edge of the pool, the sand of a beach, or a ramp to exit the water. The adrenaline will be flowing, but be sure to have your feet under you before you try to move too quickly. There will be race staff or volunteers to guide you out and toward the transition area.

Basic Technique

Technique is the key when swimming; more important than size, shape, strength, and even conditioning. Being efficient during the swim leg pays serious dividends during the bike and run segments of triathlon.

Freestyle Stroke

Freestyle, sometimes called the front crawl, is how most people naturally swim: on your stomach, reaching out with alternating hands, and pulling water back toward your sides as you rotate. Focus on mastering this technique, and don't worry about learning flip-turns right away, even while swimming in the pool. When you get to the end of the lane, just turn around and push off the wall for another lap.

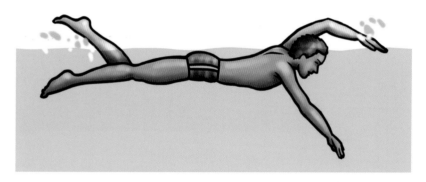

Hand entry Slice your hand in like a knife. Stab the water, make an imaginary hole in the surface, and follow your hand with the rest of your arm. Angle your hand with your palm facing inward, and lead with your little finger (like a slow-motion karate chop). The goal is to contribute to good overall hydrodynamics.

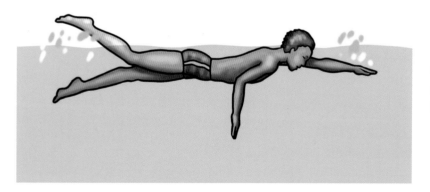

Catch Pause slightly with your arm extended as it catches and gains traction on the water.

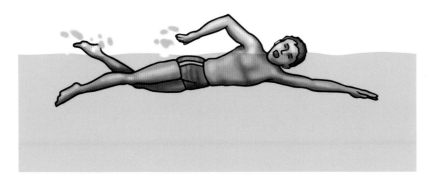

Pull Pull your hand backward along your side toward your feet, and press the water back by extending your arm to approximately 90 percent of its full extension. Be sure to keep it in line with your body to contribute to good hydrodynamics. Your arm is now ready for the recovery elbow first.

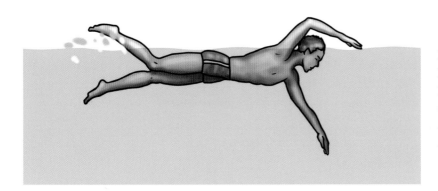

Recovery Your opposite side elbow leaves the water, with your elbow high and your hand relaxed directly under it. Your fingers trail on/near the water and then reach forward to the entry position.

A good stroke consists of reaching long, following your hand into the water, a slight pause, and then pulling the water back along your side. Be sure to keep the pull along your side. Imagine that you have two rails on either side of you to guide your arms.

Staying Long and Horizontal

As you swim, you want your body to be as horizontal in the water as possible. Swim with your head in the water, facing toward the bottom of the pool, and "pressing" down with your chest. Push your body toward the bottom of the pool. When you do these two things, your bottom half will rise and you'll increase your efficiency.

When you're swimming, you have to think l-o-n-g. Make yourself as tall as possible in the water—the greater the distance between your fingertips and your toes, the better. Imagine you're reaching for the edge of a horizontal wall with one hand. When you're fully extended, pause, and then pull yourself over it. Maximizing your reach helps you go farther with each stroke.

Focus on reducing the number of strokes you take per lap. For example, if it takes you 18 strokes to cross the pool, try to exaggerate the length of each stroke until you can gradually reduce the stroke count to below 18. You can use it as a gauge to track progress. Comparing your count from workout to workout adds motivation as you watch the number of strokes go down.

Swimming on Your Side

Swimming horizontal and swimming long both contribute to improving your hydrodynamics. The final piece is swimming on your side. This might sound confusing, but put simply: the goal is to move away from swimming flat (chest square and facing toward the bottom of the pool). Swimming like this creates drag.

Imagine reaching out with your left arm at the beginning of your stroke. You have balance in the water so you're horizontal and you're reaching long. Now begin to roll with your core/hips onto the left side of your body while you pull the water back along your right side. "Glide" on your side for a second, before you engage your core/hips and rotate to the other side. Next, reach out with your right arm, rolling to the right side of your body and pulling the water back along your left. Continue "gliding" on each side, linked by the smooth and powerful rolls. Try to aim your belly button at the sides of the pool with each turn.

It might take some time to get used to being on your side. That's normal, because it's not a natural feeling at first. But once you get comfortable there, you'll notice how effective this position can be.

Practice stealth when you swim. During your laps, listen to yourself moving through the water and focus on the noise you're making. The quieter you are, the better. If you're thrashing around, you're creating turbulence and wasting energy.

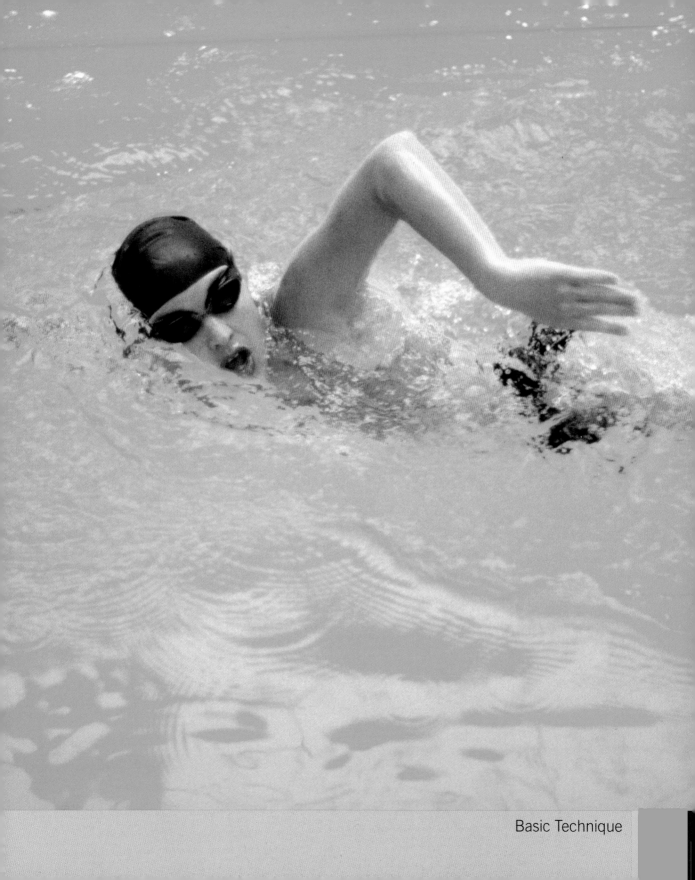

Basic Technique

Breathing and Kicking

Breathing technique is one of the most critical and sometimes intimidating elements of swimming. When you have the ability to efficiently exchange oxygen and carbon dioxide, you'll be more comfortable in the water, and as a result, better able to focus on other swimming dynamics.

Exhaling and Inhaling

In swim breathing, the exhalation occurs with a forceful blowing through the mouth. It's best to exhale underwater as you stroke; that will give you maximum time to inhale when your mouth is out of the water. If that doesn't come easily to you, you can also exhale above the water. Just keep in mind that you have limited time. When exhalation is complete, you inhale by turning your head just slightly at the top of your body rotation and sucking in all the air you can get during this brief moment when your mouth is out of the water. This movement of the head should be as subtle as possible; a simple head pivot or swivel. You will breathe in the triangle formed mid-stroke by your forearm, upper arm, and the water (almost as though you're smelling your armpit).

Bilateral Breathing

Ideally, you'll want to practice bilateral breathing: breathing to both your left and your right, as you are training and racing. Breathing only to one side can limit your perception of where you are in relation to everything else. It can also contribute to steering you off on an angle. Bilateral breathing will give you a better opportunity for a straight trajectory in the water.

Bilateral breathing is simply alternating breaths between your left and right sides. Many like to switch on the three-stroke count: left, right, left, breathe; right, left, right, breathe; and so on. However, you can change it up on the fly when you're in need of air or establish your own pattern. This type of breathing is a little more difficult than breathing to one side, but anyone at any level can learn the technique. It just takes some getting used to.

When you master breathing on both sides, you'll feel more confident in the water. It's especially handy when you're in a triathlon surrounded by other competitors. You'll take in the action on both sides of you instead of just one, improving your awareness and direction.

Additionally, this technique is extremely helpful anytime there's swell or waves hitting you from one side. You can just switch and breathe to the other side, away from the waves. Having the ability to alternate sides can be priceless in many situations.

Kicking

Many people think you have to kick like crazy to keep moving forward, but this is a misconception. Most triathletes do very little swimming with their legs. When you learn to apply the techniques outlined earlier in this chapter, you won't need to spend much energy kicking. It's very energy intensive to keep those large leg muscles moving, and the return on your effort is not very good, especially when you want to save some juice for the bike and the run.

An easy experiment will prove the truth of kicking: next time you're in the water, time how long it takes you to kick across the pool without using your arms. Then, use a pull buoy or kickboard to keep your legs afloat and time yourself using just your arms. Unless you're part dolphin, you'll probably be about two to three times faster when you use your arms.

This does not mean you shouldn't kick; just that kicking should be for assisting with your body roll while stroking, and propulsion should be secondary. Some swimmers have a natural and efficient ability to kick in conjunction with their overall swim rhythm, but focus on body roll, stroke length, balance, etc. Let your feet act as a counter balance for the body between strokes, pulls, and rolls.

Pool vs. Open Water

Depending on where you live and the time of year you are training, you may have many possible locations for swimming or you may only have one.

You can practice the same techniques in any body of water; however, those who have access to a variety of options will develop a more well-rounded experience level. Swim in as many different environments as possible. If your goal race is going to be an outdoor one, we strongly recommend that you practice swimming at least a couple times in open water. You don't want to show up at your first race in a lake or ocean without experience with oncoming waves.

Pools

Pools are great places to practice and learn proper technique. You don't need to worry about current, waves, or visibility. You can follow the black line along the pool bottom and focus on your form. Just remember: it's not how much time you log in the pool, it's the quality of that time that counts. If you're swimming 3,000 yards a day but maintaining poor technique, you won't see much improvement.

There are two main options when it comes to pool swimming: swim laps on your own or join a Masters Swim program. If possible, we recommend incorporating both into your schedule. Lap swimming is beneficial when practicing drills or your own specific training workout. Lap swim times are usually flexible, and most pools have several options throughout the day.

Masters Swim programs are simply a coached swimming experience offered at many pools and clubs. They are great because there is a sense of community and the class is goal specific. Typically, the lanes at a class are divided by skill level, with certain lanes assigned to novice, intermediate, and advanced swimmers. You might want to start in the slowest lane and advance as necessary. The coach will assign workouts, with specific goal times for each lane. The coach may also provide a critique of your form.

Be sure to follow pool etiquette. Some rules are common sense, but some are not. Consider the following next time you go for a swim:

- No diving; slide in or take the steps.

- If you're in a lane with someone else, you can split it or ask if they'd rather circle the lane.

- If you're circling in the lane, it's usually done in a counterclockwise direction (i.e., swim down the right side of the lane, turn at the wall, and swim back on the opposite side).

- If you need to pass, tap the foot of the person ahead of you once or twice to give a signal. After you hit the next wall, pass on the left.

- If you need rest, squeeze into the right corner and let others swim past you.

- Don't block any clocks swimmers might be using to track their pace or intervals.

Open Water

Open water is great for adding variety and challenge to your swim training. Whether it's in a lake, river, or an ocean, you get a whole new experience. There's no line to follow, no wall to grab, and no lane dividers. You might not even be able to see your hand when it's out extended in your stroke. At first this can be downright scary. It's okay. Hang in there. The more time you spend in open water, the more relaxed you'll become.

When swimming in open water, a wetsuit is highly recommended. It will add buoyancy and help keep you warm in colder water. In addition, you may want to tweak your technique slightly by raising your elbows a little higher than normal. This is necessary due to waves, swells, or any increase in the water's wake. Raising your elbows during the stroke helps prevent you from getting thrown off balance.

As you swim, lift your head out of the water and look forward from time to time to "sight" your surroundings. Look out for landmarks you can use to check your position while you're on the move. You don't want to lose your bearings while you're in the water.

Swimming Drills

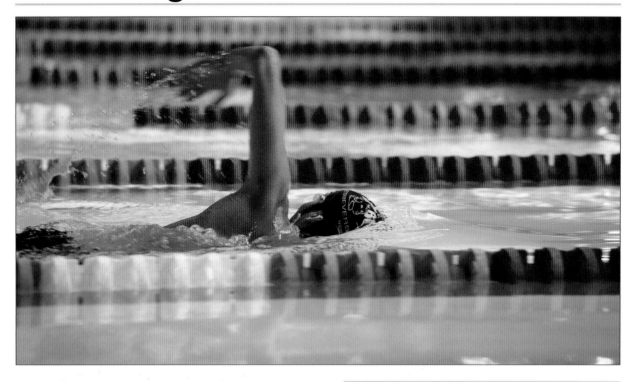

Once you have the basic stroke down, drills are great for improving your technique. Each drill builds upon the other until you have the finished product: efficient swimming. Breaking down swimming into manageable chunks is the best way to improve. When you learn one chunk, you can move on to the next. Practice these drills in the calm waters of a pool. There is no set number of times you need to do each drill.

One of the major challenges faced in swimming is overcoming oxygen debt and managing carbon dioxide levels. These drills, and swimming in general, contribute to improving your body's ability to deal with lower oxygen and higher CO_2 levels. Over time, your tolerance will develop, and you'll feel more comfortable in the water.

If you are uncomfortable in the water, take some time to get used to the pool. Try rolling on your back and floating. Spend some time underwater holding your breath. While holding onto the wall of the pool, practice bouncing above and below the surface of the water repeatedly (also known as "bobs"). This may seem very elementary, but for those who are new to the swimming, it's a good way to get accustomed to holding your breath underwater. Becoming comfortable in the water can be half the battle for many triathletes.

Swimming Drill 1: Chest Down, Butt Up

One of your major technique goals is to keep your legs from dragging as you swim. When your head is high and your butt and legs are low, you're inefficient in the water. "Chest down, butt up" will help you practice this.

Starting at the edge of the pool, push off with your face down and your arms to your sides. Use your core muscles to push your chest down and let your hips lift. The objective is to become horizontal with the surface of the water.

When you find balance, gently kick to move yourself forward. Your head is down and only lifts for air. Notice that the lower half of your body drops when you lift your head.

After you breathe, you'll regain balance and your body will begin to move back to horizontal. Return to the starting position with your chest and head down and your butt up.

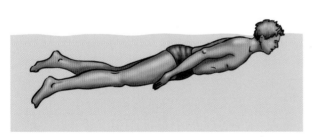

1   Begin face down with your arms at your sides.

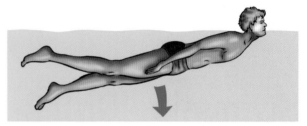

2   Your lower body drops as you lift your head to breathe.

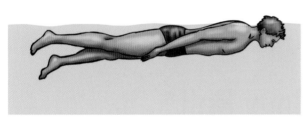

3   After you take a breath, your body should begin to move back to being horizontal.

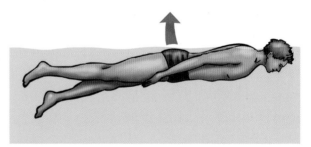

4   Concentrate on returning to the starting position, with your chest down and butt up.

Swimming Drill 2: Back Down, Butt Up

Next we'll work on learning balance from a 180-degree rotation. Take drill 1 and reverse it.

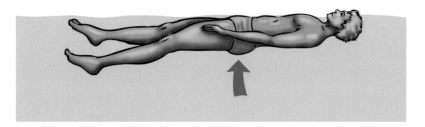

Face up with your arms to your sides. Push down through your shoulder blades. You're simulating the same balancing technique as in drill one. Gently kick yourself across the pool.

Be careful not to hit your head when you approach the wall; keep an arm above your head as you get close to it.

Swimming Drill 3: Body Roll

The body roll combines drills 1 and 2.

Start face down (head in line with your spine), arms at your sides, and kick gently. When you need air, roll onto your back. All the while, maintain balance and originate the roll with your hips so your hips, head, and torso all roll together at the same time. This establishes consistent balance. Think about it as though you are swinging a baseball bat. The swing originates with your hips and rolls through from there.

On your back, catch your breath, and roll back to your stomach. Continue doing laps in this fashion. Alternate with clockwise and counterclockwise rolls.

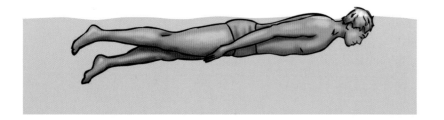

1 Head is down, arms at sides.

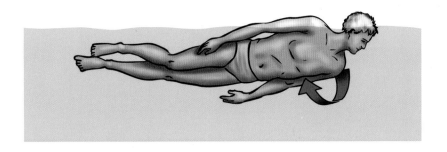

2 Roll to your back, keeping your hips, head, and torso aligned.

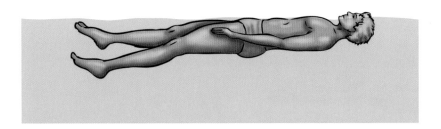

3 Take a breath while on your back.

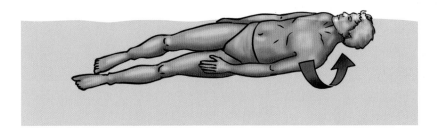

4 Roll to your stomach, keeping your hips, head, and torso aligned.

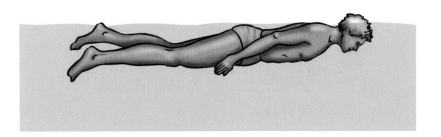

5 Return to your starting position and repeat.

Swimming Drill 4: Tall Buoy

This drill takes the "butt up" position and adds extended arms. This teaches balance in a different way by adding the element of length into the equation.

With your face down and arms out in front, kick gently across the pool. Try to only turn your head for air (don't raise your entire head). As you practice more and more with this drill, try to keep your form strong while also being able to breathe. Remember: to make your breathing more efficient, breathe out while your head is still underwater.

You will quickly notice that swimming with your arms out in front of you feels more natural than the previous drill. The long body is one that feels efficient, and allows you to glide through the water.

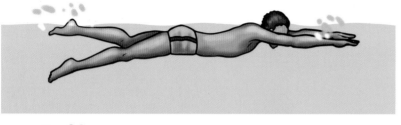

1   Begin with your face down and your arms stretched out long.

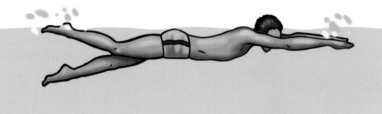

2   Kick gently across the pool.

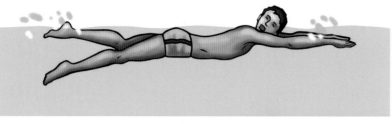

3   Turn your head for air, trying not to lift your head. Keep your hips up.

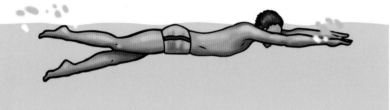

4   Return to the starting position with your face down and your arms long.

Swimming Drill 5: Sideways

Push off the wall on either side with your bottom arm extended out in front and your top arm at your side, and kick gently. Keep your face pointed toward the bottom of the pool with your cheek against your bicep. Point your belly button at the side of the pool wall. When you need air, turn your head until your mouth is just above the water line and take a breath. If you had a straight line running through your hips or shoulder blades, you'd want this line to hit the pool bottom directly underneath where you're swimming.

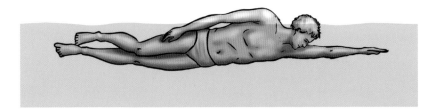

1 Keep your face down and your cheek against your bicep.

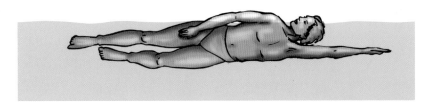

2 To take a breath, turn your head until your mouth is just above the water line.

Initially, most people will be rolled too far on their back or belly instead of exactly sideways in the water. Although it will be hard to strike the perfect balance at first, with practice this drill will really help with efficiency (alternate sides after each pool length).

In a perfect stroke, you'll end up in the "on your side" position when you're at the halfway point of each stroke. This drill will help you feel where you should end up while swimming.

Swimming Drill 6: Tall Buoy with Stroke

Incorporating all of the previous drills, we'll start to stroke with your arms, one at a time. Before one arm is able to start its stroke, you're going to wait for the first to "catch up" and touch it.

Push off the wall with your face down and arms extended, on your belly, kicking gently. When you need air, take a stroke and breathe to the stroke side at the same time. Then alternate sides. For example, when kicking along with both arms extended: pull your right arm along your side, and when it gets near your hip, roll to your side. Roll your head with your hips, take a breath, and return to the starting point (catch-up position). Then alternate sides—stroking and breathing.

This is the first drill in the progression that will give you the full stroke; all you will need to do is eliminate the "catch up."

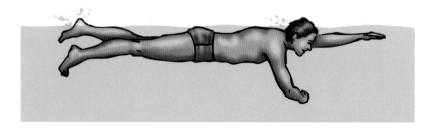

1 Begin in the Tall Buoy position.

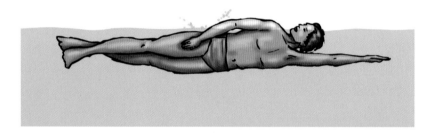

2 Begin to pull back with one arm.

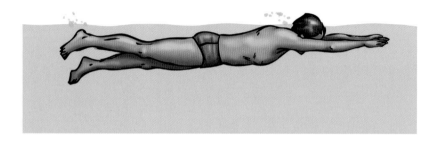

3 Rotate to the sideways postion.

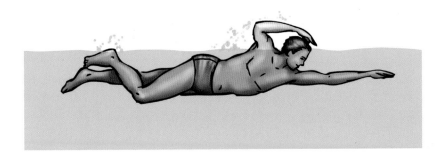

4 Stroke back toward starting position.

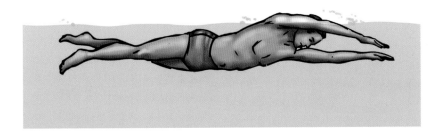

5 Complete the stroke.

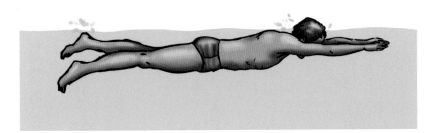

6 Return to the starting position.

As with most of these drills, this will feel awkward at first. You will want to cycle through the movements more quickly than the drill demands. Be purposeful with each stroke, and take your time.

Swimming Drill 7: Three-Count Stroke

Building on the previous drills, you'll now increase the speed of the exercise while maintaining technique. Start on one of your sides with your bottom arm extended. After a "3 count," complete half a stroke with your top arm while rolling to the center (both arms extended). Hold this position for three seconds. Repeat. Remember to keep your balance and roll your head and hips together. Breathe as needed.

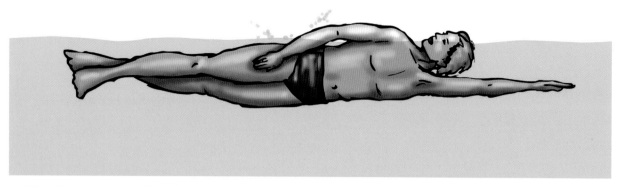

1 Begin on your side with one arm extended.

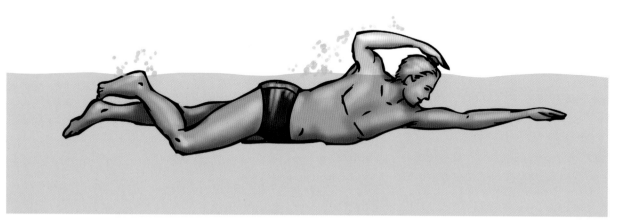

2 Count to three as you complete a half stroke with your top arm.

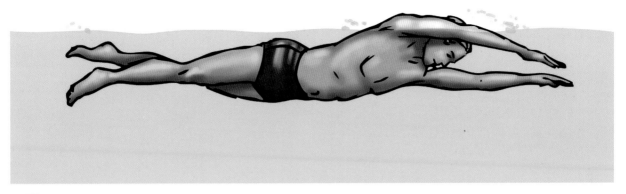

3   Roll back to the center.

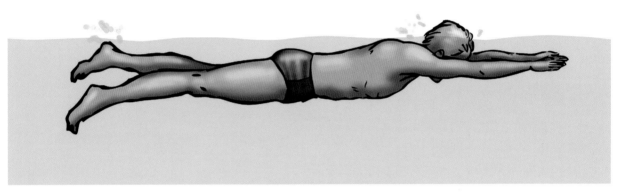

4   Hold at the center with arms and legs extended for three seconds.

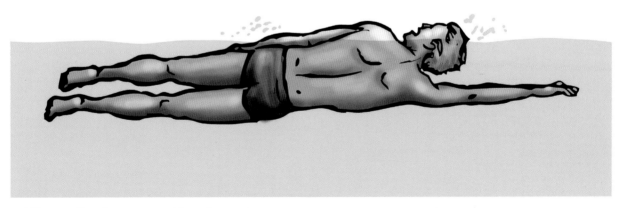

5   Roll to the opposite side and extend your top arm.

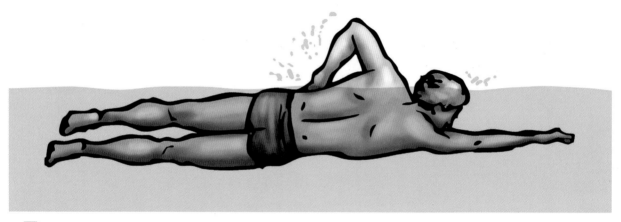

6   Count to three as you complete a half stroke.

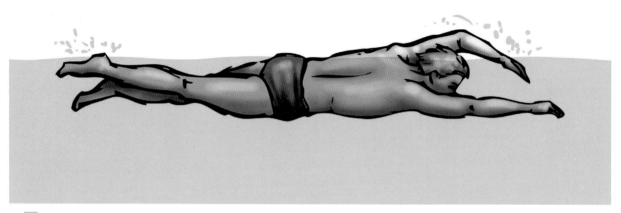

7   Roll to the opposite side and extend your top arm.

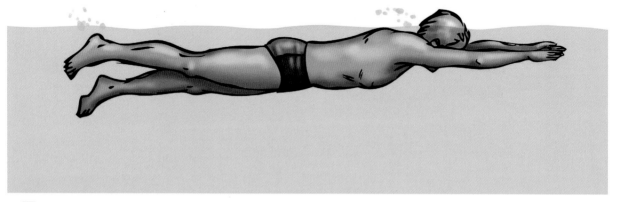

8   Hold at center with arms and legs extended for three seconds.

Swimming Drill 8: Touch Catch-Up

Drill 8 follows the same sequence of movements as drill 7. However, this time you won't do a three-second pause; you will just touch one hand to the other before pulling back. Start on one side, stroke, touch the other hand in front, pause, and pull through to the other side. Essentially, you're swimming normally with a pause out front. The catch-up gives you a reference point to return to after each stroke. Your body is rolling, and you're reaching long and pulling next to your side.

Drill Practice

Keep practicing each drill in progression. When you feel you've learned one, advance to the next. When you're confident with all eight drills, shift your goal to fine-tuning your mechanics and learning precise timing. Your objective is to maximize the force that goes into each stroke and keep momentum between strokes. When there's a good rhythm in your overall swim mechanics, your hands will move at the same rate as your body. Efficient swimming is about long glides linked by powerful rolls.

Remember:

- Press down with your chest (balance).
- Keep your head down (in line with your spine) and get air when you're in the turn.
- Originate rolls with your hips (core).
- Head, shoulders, trunk, and hips all roll together.
- Reach long and swim on your sides.
- Don't cross over the centerline of your body during your strokes.

Swim Workouts

Swim workouts might seem intimidating at first, but you will quickly realize there is nothing to fear. The suggested workouts in Part 8 of this book are laid out plainly, and you'll only need to follow along, step by step. Although you can really push it every once in a while, it is important to focus on form and technique, especially at first. The efficiencies learned and practiced will make a true difference in your time and confidence. Each workout consists of a warm-up, followed by sets of specific intervals, and concluded with a cooldown. You'll be swimming between two and four times a week, so you will have plenty of time to become acquainted with your local pool lanes.

Pool lengths are measured in either yards or meters; you can use either one for your workouts. The variance between the lengths is minimal and won't impact your training. Ideally, you want to find a pool that is long enough so you can practice drills and get into your form without constantly turning at the wall.

Swim Workout Words to Know

Intervals: Specific distances performed within a specific duration, e.g., 50 yards (or meters) on 0:55 (55 seconds).

Pace: How fast you're swimming a specific distance, e.g., 100 yards (or meters) in 1:30 (minute and a half).

Pace clock: A large clock displayed on the deck of a pool; use the clock to track both how fast you're swimming as well as rest time.

Repeats: A repetition of the distance you swim within each interval; they usually range from 25 to 800 yards (or meters).

Rest: Time taken after each interval.

Set: A series of intervals and repeats. "4×100 yd/m" is a set in which you swim 100 yard (or 100-meter) intervals, 4 times in a row.

When you see directions for a swim workout written like this ...

Swim: 3x100   2 minutes rest

... it means you're swimming 100 yards (or meters) three times, and resting for two minutes after each 100 yards (or meters).

Sample Workout

Swim:			
	Warm-up	2×100	15 seconds
	Workout	7×100	20 seconds
	Cooldown	4×50	10 seconds
	TOTAL	1,100	

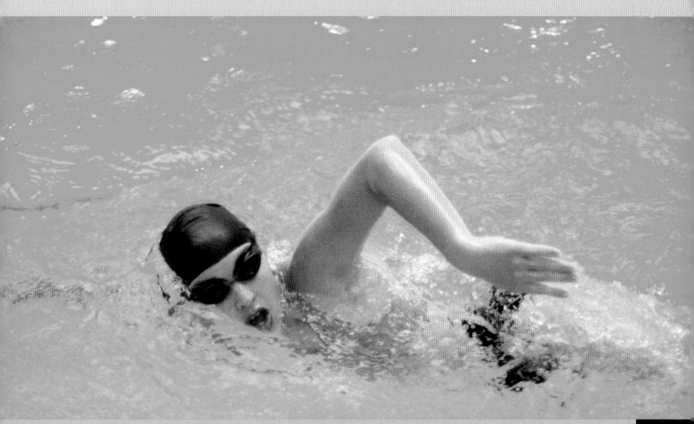

Prepare for the Unexpected

When the unexpected occurs on land, it is more or less considered part of the "norm." When the unexpected occurs in the water (e.g., a strong current starts to push you, another swimmer accidentally strikes you, your goggles become dislodged), there may be an added layer of difficulty if you can't put your feet on something solid. The key factor: DO NOT PANIC. You might find your mind playing tricks on you, and you might begin to feel panic taking over when you're in the water. Keep calm and try to relax. You may even choose to turn onto your back and float a bit, taking in some deep, cleansing breaths, or tread water. You can take that time to adjust your goggles, or just settle and regroup for a minute.

When you're swimming in open water, beware of the riptide. If there is a riptide, it is typically in the surf reports and signaled by the hazard flags on the beach from the lifeguards. If you find yourself swimming in a strong current or riptide, again: do not panic. The first instinct of many, upon realizing that they are being pulled out into the ocean, is to fight with all their might. This is the wrong response; fighting against the current will leave you quickly exhausted. Stay calm and swim parallel to the shore (perpendicular to the current) until the current subsides and then head back in. Do not attempt to fight the current head on. Taking the angled approach is much easier and safer.

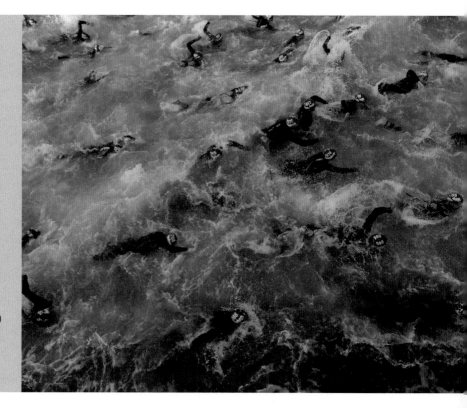

Although you won't notice yourself sweating during a swim workout, you are! Swimming burns approximately three calories a mile per pound of bodyweight. If you weigh 160 pounds and it takes you 30 minutes to swim a mile, you burn about 960 calories in an hour if your pace remains constant. Bring a bottle of water or sports drink with you to your next swim workout so you're sure to stay hydrated.

Safety Check

Use the Buddy System

Always, always, always use the buddy system when swimming in open water. Swim with at least one partner at all times. Also be sure you heed surf reports (check online, in newspapers, and on TV) and lifeguard warnings. Typically, you'll see a hazard flag flying under dangerous conditions. It's best to avoid swimming during these times.

When you go out and there's a lifeguard station, enter the water in front of the station. Tell them what you're planning to do if you're comfortable with that. At a minimum, be sure the lifeguard(s) see you go out. That way they'll know to keep an eye on you.

When you swim offshore, be mindful of how far out you go. It's better to stay in closer and swim parallel to the shore than to swim directly out into the sea. That way, you can get back to land quickly if need be.

The buddy system should apply when swimming in a pool as well. Although you don't have to bring a swimming partner with you, at a minimum be sure there is a guard or other people at the pool who would be able to assist in case of a medical emergency.

Wear Sunscreen and Lubricate

Be sure to wear waterproof or water-repellant sunscreen if you're swimming outside. Keep a bottle of spray or lotion in your swim bag at all times. Remember to reapply frequently.

Make sure to keep all of your body parts that come in contact lubricated to prevent friction. Your thighs and underarms are particularly susceptible to chafing during a swim workout. Although it is not "safety" per say, you could hurt yourself if your body cannot glide across another part of your body. Any serious chafing will make your future swimming experiences less enjoyable and more painful.

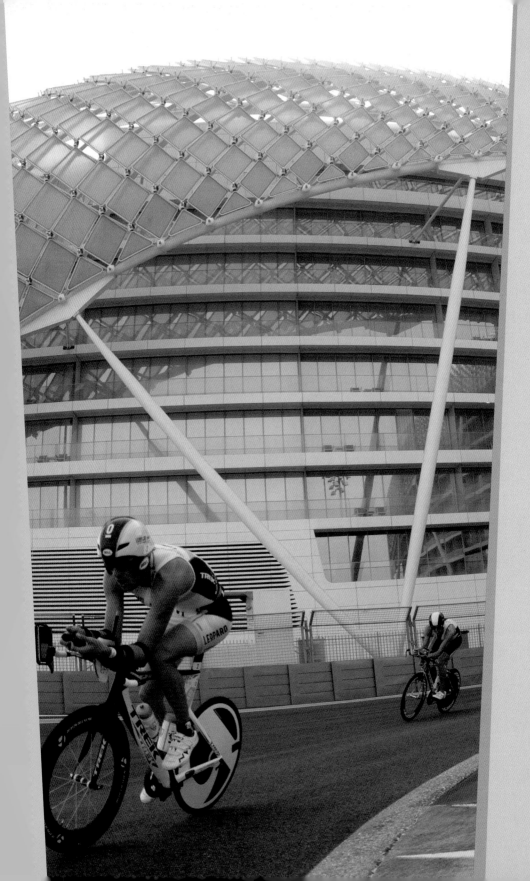

Bike

Biking is the second and longest leg of the triathlon, and the one that necessitates the most training time and gear. This part will cover the ins and outs of the bike portion of your race, from how fast you should pedal to what you should wear while doing it. You will learn the right way to prepare, train for, and race on your bike.

Many triathletes find that biking is their favorite part of training, as they get to experience their home turf with fresh eyes. Familiar streets will feel like new territory on a bike, and you'll have a reason to explore roads you haven't been down before. Although your butt might be a little sore at first, the drills and workouts outlined in this part will have you ready for your race in no time!

The Bike Stage

If you've watched triathlon on TV or been a spectator at a live event, you've seen the participants coming out of the water, getting their wetsuits stripped off, running to transition, and furiously "gearing up" in a sea of people to get on the bike course. This leg of the race may look chaotic and confusing, but it won't be if you know what to expect.

The Course

The bike course of a triathlon is typically mapped out on paved public roads that may or may not be closed to traffic. Some races may have police direct cars on one lane of a two-lane road, while the other lane is dedicated to the race. Other races may close the roads completely, and bike traffic will be just like normal car traffic.

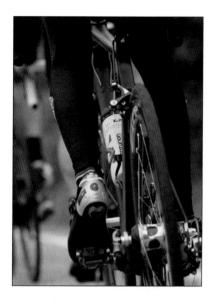

Some courses are as simple as heading out on one of side of a road, turning around at some point, and then heading back on the other side of the road. Other courses have many left and right turns, which keep you on top of your game. Depending on the distance of the bike portion of your race, you may have to do multiple loops. If this is the case, make sure you understand how to exit the course at the appropriate time.

T1: The Swim to Bike Transition

The transition area, where you swap out your gear between legs, is usually as close to the water as possible. This limits the distance that the triathletes need to run upon finishing the swim.

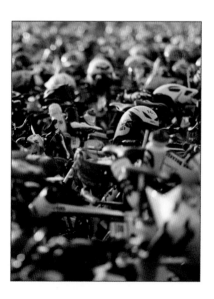

After the swim, you'll run barefooted to your bike and other gear. Watch out for rocks and try to stay calm. When you find your gear, start changing as quickly as possible. Remember to put on your helmet, as many races will disqualify participants for riding without a helmet. Additionally, make sure you cross out of the transition area (usually marked by a line across the ground or a sign) before mounting your bike.

When you first get on your bike, you're going to feel the adrenaline surging through your veins. Don't let it take over your race. When the crowd is cheering, most people will feel no pain. Check yourself, and make sure you are not pushing too hard too early.

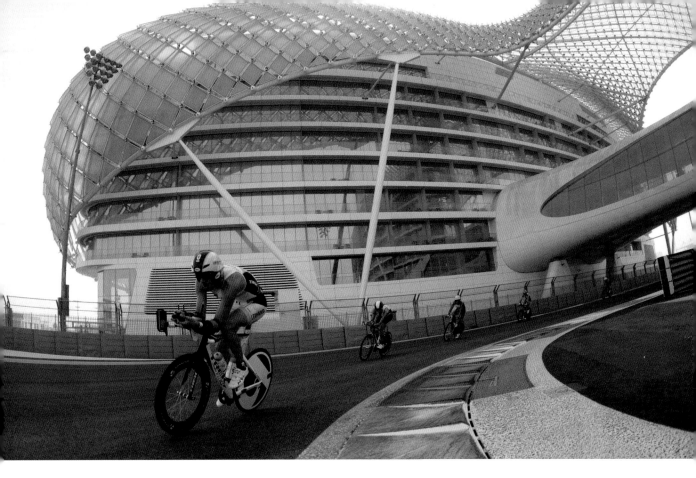

During the Ride

When you're out on the road, remember that conditions may not be perfect. It could be cold and rainy, blazing hot, or very windy. Try to ride in a variety of conditions during training, as this will help you become more prepared to face whatever happens on race day. Remember: during the race, you cannot change the conditions and everyone is dealing with them. You can do your best to control your body's reaction to adverse conditions with the appropriate gear.

Aid Stations

Depending on the length of your triathlon, there may or may not be aid stations on the bike segment of the race. Shorter triathlons usually won't provide any nutrition and will expect athletes to provide their own fuel. The information provided to you in your race packet will let you know what to expect.

Regardless of whether the race plans to supply you with some sort of food and drink, you should always plan for the worst, and at least have supplemental nutrition available, just in case. With the right preparation, the bike portion of the race will be smooth.

Getting the Right Fit

The first step in successful training for the bike portion of a triathlon is getting the proper bike fit. This process is referred to as getting "dialed in" and it ensures your comfort while riding, reduces the risk of injury, and increases your efficiency.

There are several things that can be adjusted to make the bike align to your specific body type. Start with the standard, or neutral, position and then tweak the position for comfort and aerodynamics.

If you don't feel confident setting up your bike on your own, consider working with a certified bike-fitting specialist, or someone who works at a bike shop and has experience in the matter. This may cost money, but will save you time and energy, as well as later costs associated with the aches, pains, and injuries that occur due to improper fit.

Cleat Position

If you're using clipless pedals, the first task is to screw the cleats into the correct position on the shoe. The cleat should be directly under the ball of your foot. To confirm the right spot, put on your bike shoes. Feel for the ball of your foot, and mark the spot on the exterior of the shoe with a piece of tape. Use the tape as a reference for cleat placement. A bike store employee should be able to help you with this when you're purchasing your shoes and cleats.

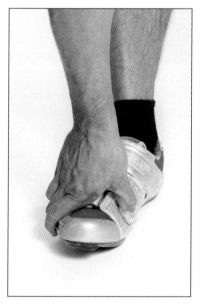
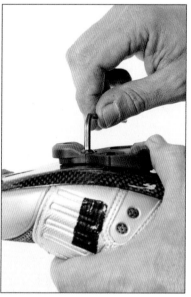
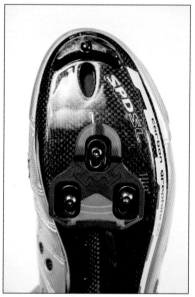

Saddle Height

For proper saddle, or seat, height, you want your leg bent at about 10 degrees when the pedal is at the lowest possible position (not quite fully extended). Make sure that your leg is just short of full extension when in the 6 o'clock position. Once it feels right, mark where the saddle stem enters the frame with masking tape. Try the bike out at this height. If you feel you are rocking side to side in the saddle when you ride, it may be too high. If you feel pain in your knee due to inadequate leg extension, it may be too low. Adjust until you find the sweet spot.

Next, adjust the saddle to maximize power. When your front pedal is in the maximum forward position, your knee should be directly above it. To check this, create a simple tool called a "plumb line." Get a string a bit longer than the length of your knee to your foot, and attach a metal nut or washer to one end. While sitting on the bike with your pedals at the 3 o'clock and 9 o'clock positions, dangle the plumb line from the side of your knee. Hold the string next to the boney knob at the head of the fibula. The string should fall right through the center of the pedal axle. If the string is in front of the axle, adjust your seat backward. If it's behind the axle, move the seat forward. Each time you adjust, recheck using the plumb line test until you are right on.

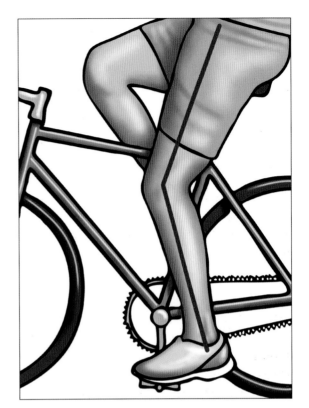

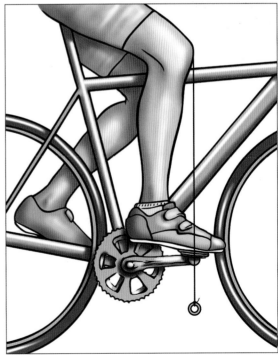

The seat and handlebars are level in neutral position.

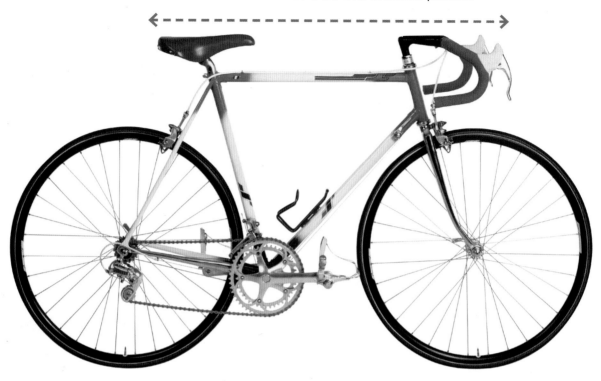

Handlebar Height

Handlebar height should be near level in relation to the saddle, the "neutral position." Use a yardstick and a carpenter's level to make your handlebars level with the saddle. Place the yardstick on the saddle and extend it toward the handlebars. Use the level to make sure the yardstick isn't tilting up or down. If the handlebars are below the yardstick, raise them until they are at the same height. If the handlebars are above the yardstick, lower them. Try riding with the handlebars in this neutral position (level with the seat) and adjust for comfort over time.

Keep in mind that the lower the handlebars are, the more aggressive the riding position is. This may be slightly more aerodynamic, but it will also put more strain on your lower back. Typically, a set-up with the handlebars level or slightly higher than the seat is more comfortable for most riders.

Using Aerobars

If you choose to use aerobars instead of regular handle bars, you can use the same method to check that they are level with the saddle. Your chest to arm angle should be about 90 degrees, with your elbow angle slightly greater. You may need to add spacers or change out your bike stem to get a comfortable fit.

When you first begin using them, aerobars, like clipless pedals, may seem awkward. Practice getting into and out of the aero position in low traffic areas when no one is in front of you. The position will feel somewhat uncomfortable initially because it changes your weight distribution (there's a shift forward in weight and balance). Another difference is that you will not have your brakes at your fingertips. Keep these things in mind and only "get aero" when you are comfortable with the road ahead.

Testing Your Fit

After you have the right bike fit, you will want to test these elements on a ride. Determining where to ride will be influenced by your abilities and confidence. Safety is the first priority when riding—the less traffic, the better. Find the safest roads you can, and be aware of your surroundings.

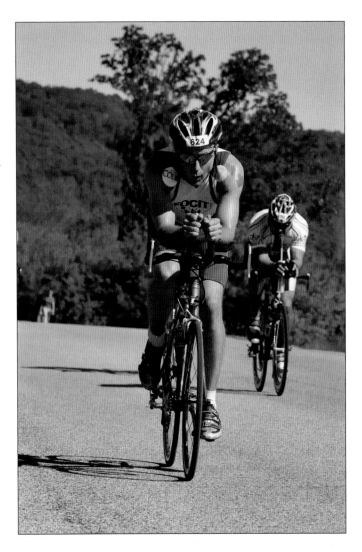

Biking Basics

Compared to to running, the bike ranks really well on the low-impact activity index (swimming is still less impact). Your upper body carries very little load except for supporting its own weight. If you use aerobars, you can even transfer that weight from a muscle-bearing load to a skeletal-bearing load (in other words, your bones will support your upper body with almost no energy expended). The lower body takes on some force through the ankles, knees, and hips, but good form can help reduce overall impact and possibility for injuries.

The Importance of Form

In a triathlon, the bike segment is between the swim and the run. When you get off the bike, you'll need to have enough energy left to conquer the run. The way to ensure this happens is to practice good technique. Proper form reduces the amount of energy expended, and the less energy expended on the bike means more energy for the run.

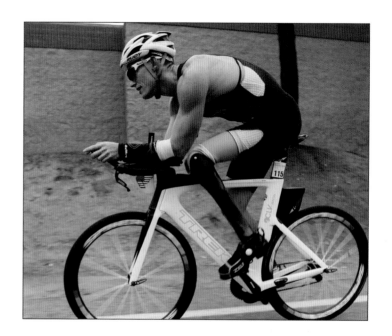

Ideally, when you cycle, you want to have a "quiet" upper body. This means it shouldn't move much, and should be still and relaxed. Your upper body should be used for balance, steering, and to grab your water bottle or fuel when necessary. Let the legs and lower body handle the work. Some people think the quadriceps or thighs handle most of the effort, but in reality, when practicing good form, you'll work quadriceps, hamstrings, calves, and the strongest muscle in the body—the gluteus maximus.

Where to Ride

The type of terrain on which you ride affects how your cycling legs will develop. If you ride hills, you'll build stronger legs more quickly than you would from riding on level ground. You'll work harder on the hills, but will get a respite on your way down. When you climb and recover, you are doing a form of interval training. Riding on level ground, or flats, also has its challenges. Your power output may be less on the flats, but you'll probably be keeping a constant pace with little opportunity to coast and take a break. If you live in an area where it is possible, we recommend training on all types of terrains.

Some cities have bike lanes on several roads, and if you're lucky enough to have them in your area, take advantage. These provide a specific lane for bikes, and give you space that should help buffer you from other traffic. Keep in mind that you still need to be vigilant in your travels.

Another option may be bike paths. These are typically located in a park or forest preserve, and therefore shut off from most vehicular traffic. These are great because you don't need to worry about traffic and intersections; you can just focus on your form and ride.

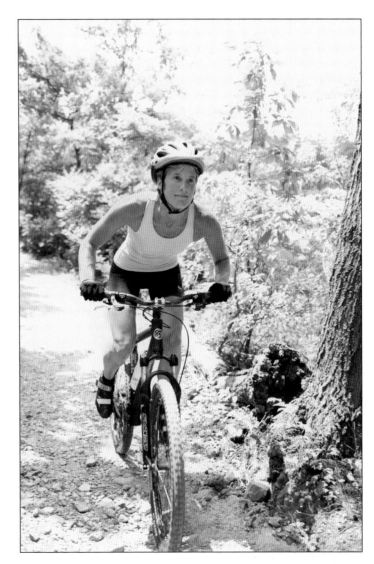

Pedaling, Pacing, and Cadence

In addition to having a bike that fits properly and practicing good form, the specifics of your body mechanics have to be honed in order to achieve peak performance. Paying attention to your pedaling, pacing, and cadence will help you minimize energy expenditure.

Pedaling

Most people are used to bikes with standard flat pedals, and they push "down" to move. However, when you only push down and do not exert any upward force, you are greatly limiting your potential power and increasing your fatigue.

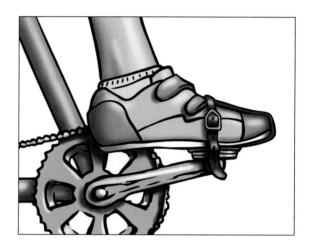

We highly recommend using toe clips, pedal straps, or clipless pedals to secure your feet to the pedals. Good technique on the bike centers on the "full circle" mentality. You shouldn't just push down with one leg and then wait for the pedal to rotate around before pushing down again. Instead, you exert force throughout the rotation.

If you're new to the clipless system, do not head straight onto the roads. Find a spot where you can hold yourself upright on your bike without moving (perhaps in a doorframe), and practice clipping in and out of your pedals. This will get you used to the motion. Once you have those mechanics down, you can try it while moving.

Spend some time riding in a large area that has no traffic, such as an off-hours parking lot. Practice clipping in and out of the pedals until it becomes second nature. This will help avoid anxiety and falls later while you're in the middle of an intersection.

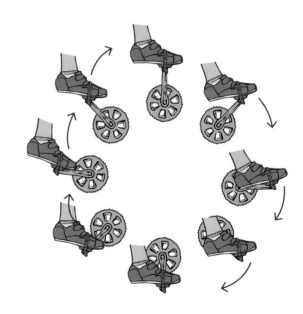

You can also improve efficiency with your "line," the path your bike takes. Even when riding straight, many cyclists make tiny corrections that cause their bikes to swerve slightly, which increases the distance the tires are covering. To avoid over-correcting, keep your focus a bit ahead of you.

Cadence

In cycling, cadence refers to revolutions per minute (RPM), or how many times your pedals go around in one minute. You can determine your cadence while riding by counting the number of times your right knee rises for ten seconds and multiplying by six. On flat ground, the optimal range is between 80 and 100. Cycling downhill will raise your cadence, while cycling uphill will probably lower it (although shifting gears will compensate for some of that).

In order to achieve the ideal cadence range (80–100 RPMs), you must shift gears with some regularity. If you have "drop" style handlebars with the shifter right next to the brake, you'll be able to smoothly shift as necessary when in the drops. If you have aerobars with shifters at the tip of the bar, or a shifter on the frame, it will be slightly more effort to reposition your hands and keep your cadence steady. You'll learn to transition between shifting and your regular and/or aero riding position.

Most riders do not shift enough. This leads to inconsistent cadence and effort. It takes practice to learn the gears, find your RPM range, and maintain desired intensity zones. Using a bike computer or biking app on your phone is an easy way to keep track of your cadence.

Pace

Your pace, or speed, depends on the purpose and duration of the ride. Different types of rides require different speeds. If it's an easy training day, your pace may be slower than normal. If you're racing in a sprint-distance triathlon, your pace may be near maximum effort. If you're training in an interval group bike class (such as a Spinning® class), your pace may vary from easy to intense. Pacing is an important component of the bike discipline, and can be difficult to master at first. Know yourself, your goals, and your race. It's easy to get caught up in what someone else is doing and fall out of your intensity zones. It happens. When it does, refocus on your RPM, intensity, and overall status. Make adjustments as needed, but find *your* pace.

Fueling Your Body

Of the three disciplines, the bike is the most important for fueling (ingesting calories and hydrating) during a race. It's the longest segment, and your upper body is relatively motionless, making it easier to take in and digest fuel. You can replenish the calories you lost while swimming and those you're burning in the moment, and you can pack a little reserve for the run.

What Is "Fuel"?

"Fuel" comes in many forms. You can choose from a wide variety of products specifically designed to be consumed during endurance sports, but you can also get fuel from everyday grocery store items. Most of the products on the market contain sugar, salt, and caffeine and are meant to provide calories and nutrients that are easily assimilated by your body. This fuel will keep you going, boost your performance, and balance electrolytes.

Some of these products include:

- Powders that can be added to your sports drink or water to give you extra calories.
- Gels in small packets that are easy to open and swallow on the move.
- Chewy gummy candies and jelly beans fortified with sodium and potassium for electrolyte balance.

Regular grocery store foods can be used, too. Honey, fruit leather, bananas, pretzels, breakfast pastries, cola, and energy drinks are common choices.

How to Fuel

During a race, you must take in nutrition while maintaining a straight pace line, avoiding road hazards, and navigating through other competitors and vehicles. Similar challenges exist when you're out for a training ride. The best advice is to slow down, coast, keep an eye on the road, and slowly ingest the food or drink. One hand near the stem offers more steering stability while you're negotiating your nutrition (but also takes your hands away from your brakes).

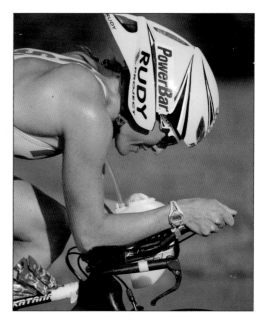

When you're out for a training ride, you'll either have to bring your fuel with you or be prepared to purchase it along the way. Where you store your fuel is a matter of personal preference.

Many people pack their nutrition bars, gels, and other supplements in their jersey pockets. While out riding, it is not too difficult to just reach back and retrieve a gel, tear it open with your teeth, and ingest some tasty and necessary calories.

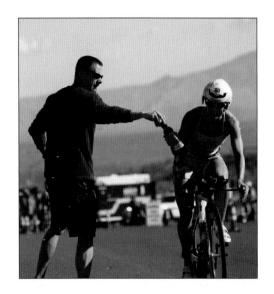

The important thing is that you can easily access your fuel without interrupting your ride. Make notes after a training session on your nutrition strategy. Once you find something that works, you'll be that much closer to getting to the finish line with a smile.

Many races will have aid stations along the way. They will usually have options like water, sports drink, energy gels and bars, and maybe even bananas. When approaching the aid station, if you intend on grabbing something from one of the volunteers, move safely toward the side the aid station is on. Don't be afraid to slow down. As you reach out to grab your nutrition, keep your arm loose. Grab the nutrition and let your arm swing back. Once it is in your hand, eat it or put it away as soon as possible, and get your hands back on the handlebars!

When to Fuel

If you're going right into biking or running after a swim workout, we recommend easing into the fuel. Try not to eat too much too fast right out of the water. Have a gel or some other soft food waiting for you; don't try to consume an entire nutrition bar. Hopefully you won't have any trouble, but be cautious in the transition after a swim. Give your body a chance to acclimate from horizontal swimming to a completely different movement.

When you're out on the road, you should try to eat a little bit at a time. At a minimum, you should try to have a little snack every 30 minutes or so. If you're using a powder mixed with your drink, keep drinking on a regular basis to ingest your fuel.

During the ride, the promise of a specific tasty treat is a great way to stay motivated. We like to eat something special at the halfway point or toward the end of a ride because it gives us something to look forward to.

The bottom line is that nutrition is of great importance and specific to the individual. Practice with various strategies during your training so you are ready to implement them on race day.

Outdoor Training

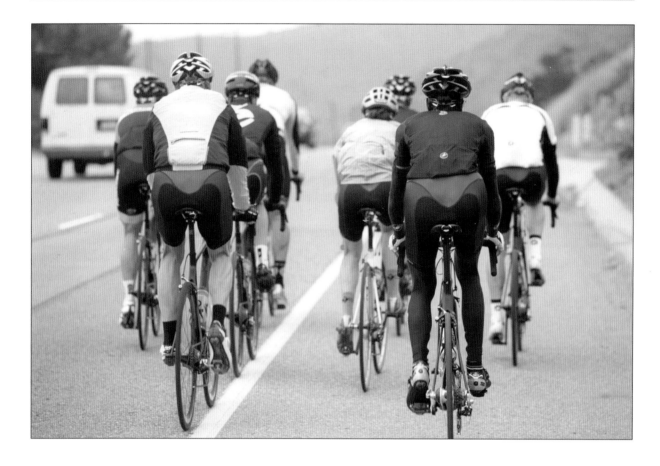

When you ride your bike on the road, you have the same rights and share the same responsibilities as other vehicles. On your bike, you are less visible than a car, so you need to be extra attentive to traffic and everything around you beyond those driving.

The duration, intensity, and terrain of your rides will vary depending upon your goals and your environment, and you should plan to incorporate variety in your training.

Most beginners doing a short race will be able to train for the bike portion of the triathlon simply by riding several miles per week. If you want to do more than just put miles in, there are different ways to challenge yourself on outdoor rides.

Terrain

Once you're comfortable riding on flat and rolling terrain, you may want to challenge yourself with more difficult rides. Steeper hills help improve muscular strength and endurance. They give you an opportunity to stand up from time to time, recruit more muscle groups, and stretch out a little. In addition to the physical benefits of climbing, you'll also appreciate the change of scenery.

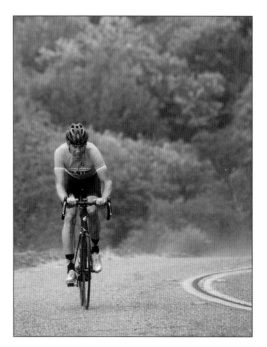

To really push yourself, consider hill repeats. All you need to do is find a longer hill, climb up, come back down, and repeat. Set a goal for the number of repeats you'd like to accomplish, and see if you can do it. You may want to keep track of how long each climb takes you, and see if you can keep that number steady. As always, keep an eye out for traffic and make sure you start braking early enough on your descent to stay safe.

Wind and Weather

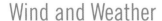

Training outside means you have to contend with weather conditions, and the most important thing to consider about weather is to put your safety first. Generally, it isn't recommended to train in the rain, but if it starts to rain while out on a ride, you need to know what to do. With rain, like darkness, drivers will not be able to see you as easily. If there is a chance visibility will get bad during your ride, clip a red flashing light on the back of your jersey. If there is lightning, you should reschedule the ride.

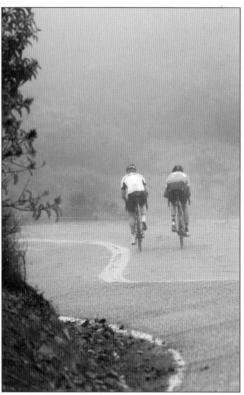

There are a couple other things to consider if riding in the rain:

1. You will immediately become wet, which can drop your body temperature. Think about wearing a waterproof jacket

2. Traction will be worse than normal. Be especially careful riding across leaves, on painted lines on roads, and railroad tracks. When riding over these things, try to keep your line straight (don't attempt to turn unless you need to).

Riding into a strong headwind or a crosswind will make your ride harder, but is a good experience to have while training. When it happens, stay calm and do your best to stay in your line. Don't fight the wind too much; it's okay if you get blown a little. If you lean into the wind too much and the gale dies abruptly, you might overcompensate and get out of control. If you have aerobars, now is the time to use them. If not, lower yourself into the drops (the lower part of standard handlebars).

High heat? No problem. Just make sure to stay hydrated throughout your ride. If you have limited water bottles on your bike, make sure you will be passing somewhere that you can fill up during the ride.

With proper clothing and equipment, adverse weather conditions will only improve your training. When your race day comes, you'll be ready for anything.

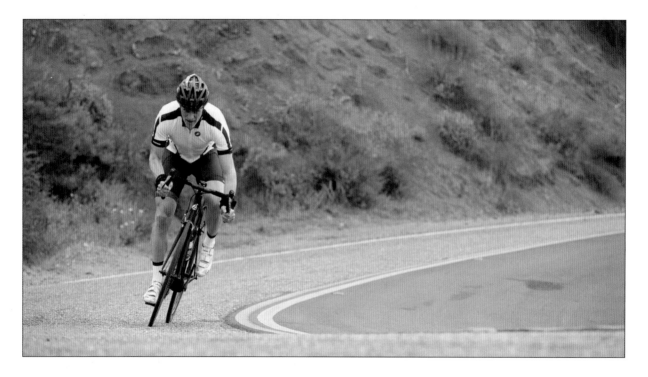

Turning

Knowing how to turn properly is critical, especially at higher speeds, and on hilly terrain. When you're heading into a sharp turn, brake before the turn. To stay in control, gradually apply your brakes prior to the turn, rather than fully squeezing your brakes at the last second. If the grade of the hill is very steep, most of the braking should be done using the rear brake. Additionally, when you are heading into a sharp turn, always keep your inside leg up and the outside leg down. This will help in balance and in keeping your foot from catching the ground as you lean into the turn.

Race Preparation

For race preparation, it is always best to train on roads that resemble the course of your future race. To get a feel for the course, read information posted on the event's website or consider contacting the race director. Established events often have online forums where triathletes who have raced the course in the past will post about their experiences. The more information you have, the more you can tailor your training.

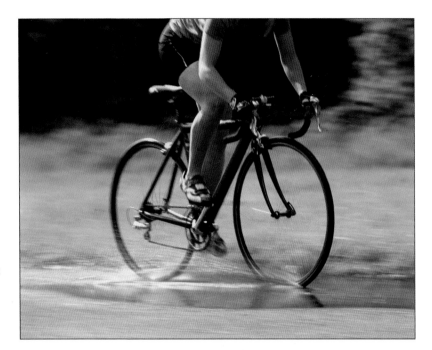

Tips for Riding

- If you're approaching a bump in the road, lift yourself up off your saddle so you can absorb the impact with your arms and legs (not your butt).

- Keep your fingers loose. This helps reduce wasted energy in your hands.

- If your feet start to tingle or burn, wiggle your toes and check that your shoes are not too tight. You may be experiencing poor circulation.

- When you first start cycling, you may notice your butt getting sore from the saddle. Don't worry; it will get better over time, as that area becomes "conditioned."

Indoor Training

There will be times when weather, traffic, or road conditions will require you to take your bike training indoors. Some popular choices for indoor training include stationary bikes, bike trainers, and group classes.

Stationary bikes are good if you're in a pinch. The downside is that they don't have the same geometries as your personal bike. Drastic changes in the bike set up can lead to injury, so try to use them sparingly if possible.

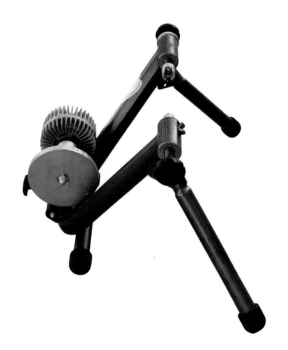

Bike trainers are great because you can set them up with your own bike. This maintains consistent biomechanics with your outdoor riding. Some trainers just elevate your back wheel, add resistance, and allow you to spin indoors, while higher-end models include computers that measure watts, speed, and cadence.

A **group exercise class** like Spinning® can add extra motivation and a social aspect to your workouts. These are led by an instructor and each session has a specific goal, such as focusing on endurance or intervals.

These drills can be done using a bike trainer or other indoor cycle bike. For each drill, begin with an easy 10-20 minute warm-up and finish with a 10-20 minute cooldown.

Indoor Bike Drills

Single Leg Drills (SLDs)

Sit on the bike and clip one cleat into the pedal. Leave the other cleat out of the pedal and rest it on a box or table, out of the way of all moving parts. Remember to keep the rest of your body in normal riding line; you don't want the one leg off the bike to throw you out of balance.

Start pedaling in a very easy gear using the one leg. This is the time to really hone in on the technical aspect of your riding.

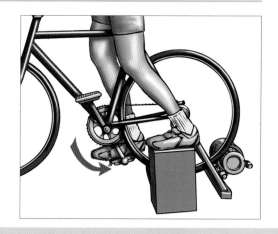

Focus on the full circle and make things as smooth as possible while keeping the RPM above 80. You can shift as needed.

Start spinning with the one leg for 30 seconds, then clip in the second leg and use both to recover for 15 seconds.

Finally, unclip the first leg and switch to second to complete the first interval. Repeat the interval four or five times. As you progress in training, add duration to each repetition and repetitions to each set.

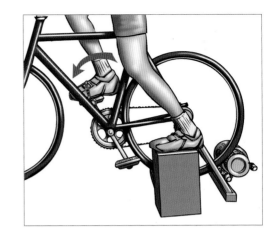

Large Gear Drills (LGDs)

LGDs are performed using both legs in a large gear and at a lower RPM. These intervals are great for increasing muscular strength and muscular endurance. The idea is analogous to weight lifting: the drill is more focused on muscular fitness than cardiovascular endurance. Stay seated, keep it smooth, and focus on the circular motion of each pedal stroke.

Spin in a larger gear for two minutes (less than 80 RPM); recover for one minute in an easy gear (less than 100 RPM); then repeat intervals three to five times.

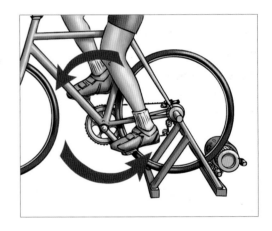

Small Gear Drills (SGDs)

SGD are again performed using both legs and will really get your legs spinning fast. These speed intervals help develop your neuromuscular system by teaching it to fire efficiently at higher rates. While doing these drills, it's very important to maintain good form. If you begin to bounce in the saddle, slow it down. Focus on applying consistent force all the way around the pedal stroke. You will want to spin very fast, but if your form starts to suffer, get into a slightly harder gear and back down the RPMs a tad.

Spin at a high RPM (greater than 100) in an easy gear for 60 seconds and then recover for 30 seconds. Repeat this four to five times. The goal of this speed interval is to pedal as fast as possible while maintaining good form.

Basic Bike Maintenance

Owning a bike means you will have to perform basic maintenance activities such as taking it apart for traveling, oiling the chain, and changing flat tires. Learning to do these things on your own will save you time, money, and frustration down the road. In addition, at a minimum, you should get your bike professionally tuned at the beginning of the season. You might consider taking it in again a week or so before a big race.

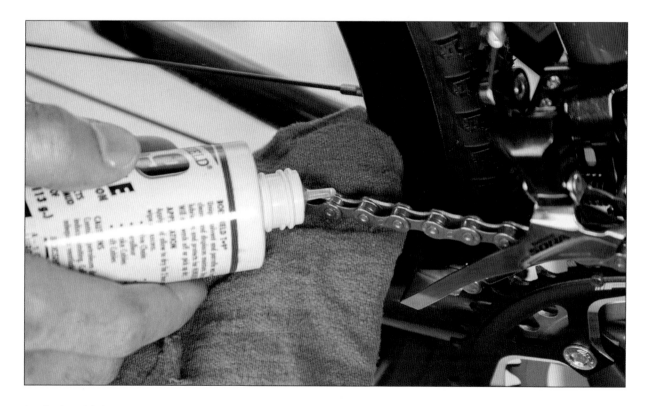

Lubrication

Keep your bike clean and the chain lubricated. Purchase a good degreaser from an auto parts or bike shop to help with cleaning the chain and anything else that may be greasy. One way to clean your chain is to wet a rag with a degreaser, lightly grip the chain with the rag, and then turn the pedal backwards. Turn the pedals enough times so that the chain makes a full rotation, and that each link of the chain slides through the rag between your fingers. Use an old toothbrush to get hard to reach areas such as chainrings (gears). After the chain is clean, you'll want to reapply some lubrication. There are several types and brands of lube available. It comes down to price and preference. You may want to try a couple different products to find your favorite.

Bike Valves and Tubes

There are two kinds of valves for bicycle tubes: a Presta, or European valve, is long and skinny and is usually used on road bikes; a Shrader, or American valve, looks like a car tire's valve and is usually used on older model bikes. Some of the Presta valves are longer than others to accommodate a specific rim. Tire and tube sizes will also vary from bike to bike. There are different dimensions. Sometimes the numbers appear in millimeters and sometimes in inches. We recommend writing your size down or taking an old tube to the bike shop when getting a replacement.

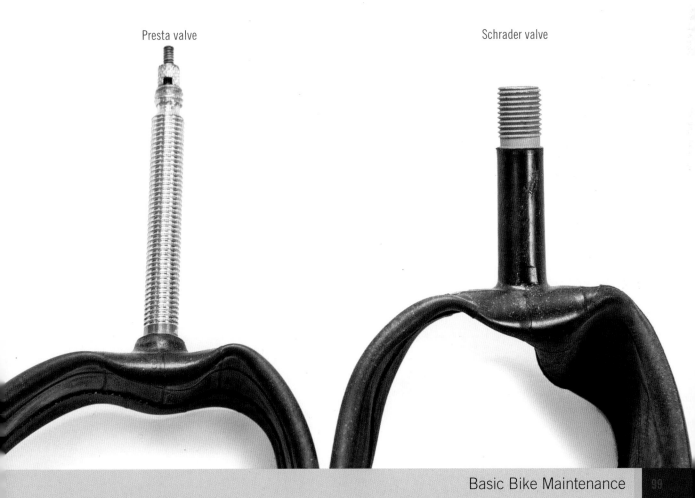

Presta valve

Schrader valve

Flat Tires

Flat tires are inevitable. If you're riding on clincher tires, which have tubes and are the easiest type to repair on the road, follow these steps to replace the punctured tube. For tubular tires, which have the tube sewn into the tire, talk to your local bike shop expert to discuss changing a flat for your specific type of wheel. If you've never changed a flat before, practice doing it at home first.

Changing a flat front tire is less involved but otherwise the same as changing the back. Here's how to change a flat back tire.

1. Shift gears so that the back gear is on the smallest ring. This will make it easy to replace the chain when you put the tire back on.

2. Loosen the skewer (the bike's axle) and take the wheel off the frame. (For the back wheel, this will involve some maneuvering with the chain and gears.)

3. Using the tire valve, release the remaining air from the tire.

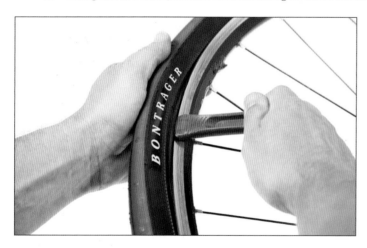

4. Insert the flat end of a tire lever (a shoe horn for your tire) between the rim and the tire.

5. Push the other end of the lever down until there's a gap between the rim and the tire, and hook the lever onto a spoke.

6. Place the flat end of the second tire lever into that gap, and start sliding it around the rim.

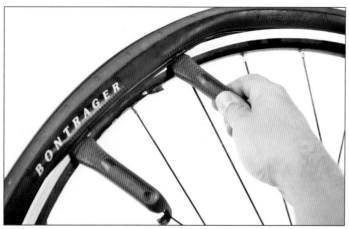

7. Work the second lever all the way around the full tire until it's back near the first lever and one full side of the tire is off the wheel.

8. Leaving one side of the tire on the rim, pull the old tube out starting directly opposite the valve. (Put the tube in a back jersey pocket to patch or discard later.)

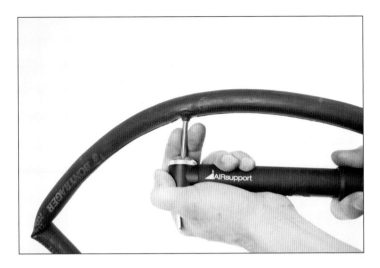

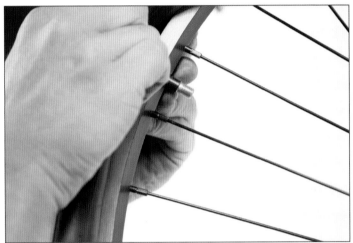

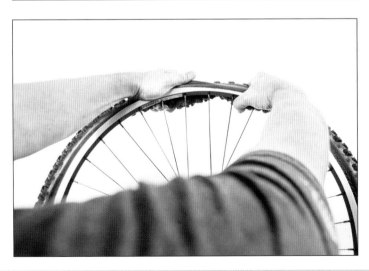

9. Gently run your fingers along the inside of the tire to locate any potential causes of the flat.

10. Pump a couple of strokes of air into the new tube to make the refitting easier.

11. Begin putting the new tube on the wheel and under the tire by inserting the valve through the hole in the rim. Using both hands, fit the tube around the rim, working your way from the valve in both directions. (Don't let the tube become pinched between the tire and rim.)

12. Starting at the valve stem, begin pushing the tire back on the rim by hand, and work your way from that spot in both directions.

13. When the tire gets taut toward the end, use the heel of your palm to push the remaining part of the tire over the rim. You may need the tire lever to pop it into place. (Be careful not to pinch the tube.)

14. Push the valve stem up into the tire to clear any part of the tube that might have been caught, and then pull it back down.

15. Inflate the tire using your pump or CO_2 cartridge.

16. Remount the wheel.

Prepare for the Unexpected

Of the three sports in a triathlon, biking involves the most complex piece of equipment and therefore has the greatest opportunity for mechanical failure. Extra planning is necessary when going out on training rides and on race day to be ready for anything.

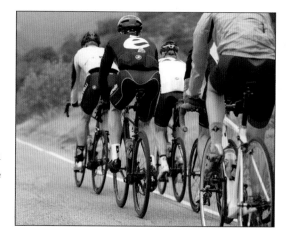

When training, it's good practice to ride with a buddy or in small groups, so if something does go wrong, you've got back up. There are going to be times when you forget to bring something important along on your ride, and if you are alone, you could end up pushing or carrying your bike back to civilization. It's also great for camaraderie and sharing biking and triathlon tips.

If you do ride alone, you absolutely must take a cell phone with you. Put it in your saddle bag or back jersey pouch and only use it if you have to. Don't talk on the phone while riding.

Safety Check

Above all, train safe. Biking involves moving parts, unknown road conditions, and high speeds. You can get into precarious situations if you're not careful. Stay vigilant, and you'll be fine.

Items for the Road

- Saddle bag or other storage pouch
- Cell phone*
- Spare tube(s)*
- Tire levers (two or three)
- Frame pump or CO_2 cartridges*
- CO_2 valve adapter (if using cartridges)

- Multi-purpose compact bike tool (contains Allen wrenches, screw drivers, etc.)*
- Cash*
- Water bottle(s) and cages or hydration system*
- Energy bars/gels or other nutrition

- Map of the area
- Sunglasses*
- Helmet*
- Gloves
- Cycling jersey and shorts
- Bike shoes and socks

*Critical item

On the Road

Keep an eye out for sewer grates. Some grates may run parallel to your bike's tire path and your tire could fall into the gaps. Cattle grates typically run perpendicular to the flow of traffic, and you can safely ride over them. At railroad tracks, use common sense and caution. Check for a train and then ride with care over the tracks, making sure to keep your tires perpendicular to the tracks.

Always stay in control while riding, and don't let your riding exceed your ability. Don't ride on narrow paths where you need to keep your wheels within a limited space, and don't fly down hills if you will have to stop or take a corner at the bottom.

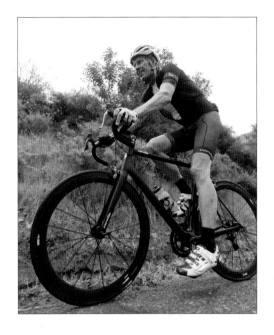

Night and Rain Riding

Darkness magnifies all of the safety issues riders face during the day, so illuminating yourself and your path are the priorities. Wear reflective tape, lights, and reflectors. Helmet-mounted headlights provide light on what you're gazing at, and bike-mounted lights will give you additional, steady light. Keep a backup battery with you, too.

Clear protective eyewear is also essential while riding at night. It protects you from wind and anything airborne, such as dirt or bugs that could fly into your eyes.

Riding in the rain or on wet roads is not recommended either. Pavement lines can be extremely slippery, especially on turns, and drivers will have reduced visibility. Wear a light on your back, and some sort of protective eyewear. After riding in the rain, dry your bike as soon as possible to prevent rust.

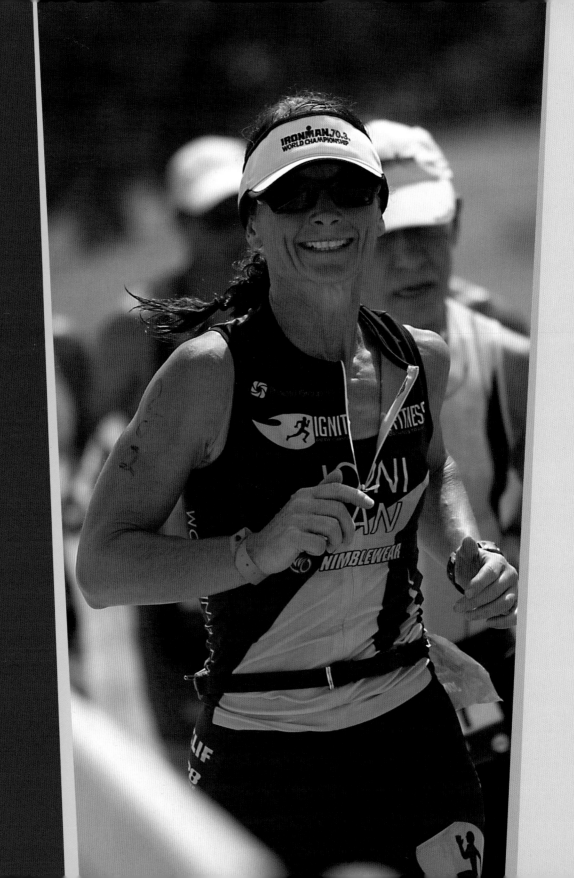

Run

Running is a superb cardiovascular exercise that requires very little gear. Few other fitness activities elevate your heart rate as effectively and consistently as running. Running improves your cardiovascular fitness, which in turn strengthens your overall health.

This part provides the information and strategies you need to successfully train for and complete the last leg of your triathlon. If you're already a runner, you might know some of the information and have some of the gear, but this part will get you prepared for the run portion of your race.

If the thought of running scares you, be aware that many triathletes do a run/walk combo throughout their training and during their actual race. Whatever your pace, the drills and workouts outlined in the upcoming sections will have you prepared to finish your race strong.

PART 5

The Run Stage

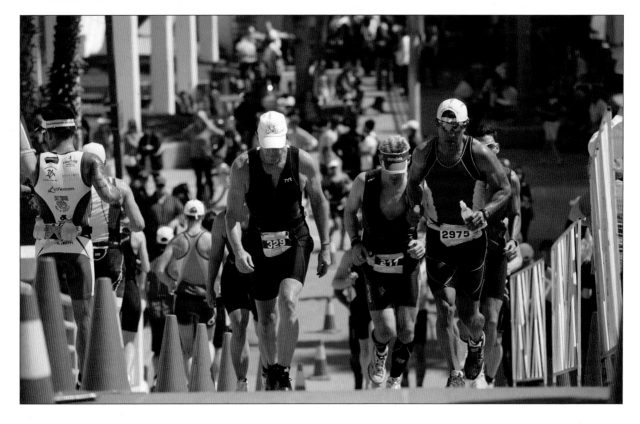

The running portion of a triathlon looks a lot like a typical road race. It can be crowded, but unlike biking and swimming, you won't have water or wheels to contend with. The more familiar you are with the logistics of the run portion of the race, the more comfortable you'll be with what lies ahead.

T2: The Bike to Run Transition

The "bike to run" transition (T2) area will almost always be the same as the "swim to bike" transition (T1) area. After the bike portion, you'll run your bike back to your other gear and put it on the rack. Stay calm and composed. Switch out your shoes, ditch your helmet, and swap out any other necessary gear.

Just like your first transition (T1), you're going to feel the adrenaline pumping when you first run out onto the course. Don't let it take over your race. Do not push too hard too early, as you will end up suffering later. Let your legs and feet acclimate to the new motion and the road. It is always better to go slowly at the beginning and push yourself hard as you get toward the end of the race.

Location

The run portion of the triathlon most often takes place on city roads, but might also be through parks or forest preserves, or even on a beach. If the race is out on the road, it will almost always be shut down by police. On trails, you may or may not encounter people not in your race. Just keep your head up and be aware of what is going on around you.

Course Layout

Some courses are as simple as heading out on one side of a road, turning around at some point, and then heading back on the other side of the road. Other courses have many left and right turns through city blocks, which keep you alert. If your run includes multiple loops, make sure you understand how to exit the course at the appropriate time.

Aid Stations

Depending on the length of your triathlon, there may or may not be aid stations on the run segment of the race. For shorter triathlons, athletes are often expected to provide their own fuel. Check your race packet for aid station information and come prepared.

Regardless of whether fuel will be supplied during the race, you should always plan for the worst, and at least have supplemental nutrition available for yourself in the transition area. When you get off your bike, you'll probably be ready for a snack. Have a bite as you're changing, or bring it out on the course with you.

With the right preparation, the run portion of the race will be smooth.

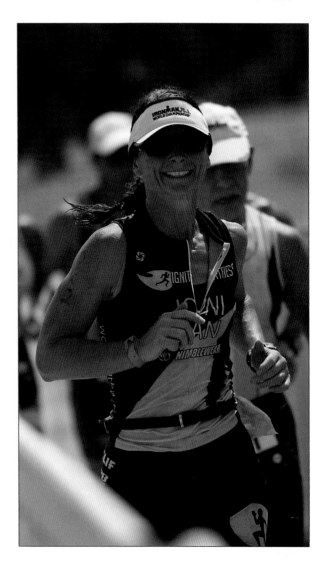

Running Basics

Running is the perfect fitness exercise because location is not a limiting factor. People can run anywhere in the world as long as it's safe. If it's hot, bring some water with you; if it's cold, dress in layers; if there are a lot of hills, go slower and take smaller steps than you would on flat terrain.

If running seems a little overwhelming at first, it's okay to walk. Especially in the beginning of your program, you might walk some or most of the minutes in your "run" workout. Slowing to a walk during a running workout isn't cheating. Almost all runners walk from time to time; it's a great way to break up the work into smaller pieces. In fact, walking can and should be used as part of the warm-up, cooldown, and in between.

Technique

When running, you want to keep your feet landing slightly in front of you, and relatively close to your body's centerline. Keeping your feet landing on or near the centerline helps you in two ways: it creates less stress on your knees, hips, and ankles, and it keeps you from wasting energy on side-to-side movement. If you're not sure how your form stacks up, ask a friend to photograph or record your stride while on a treadmill or out on a sidewalk. You'll quickly see if you're landing near the centerline.

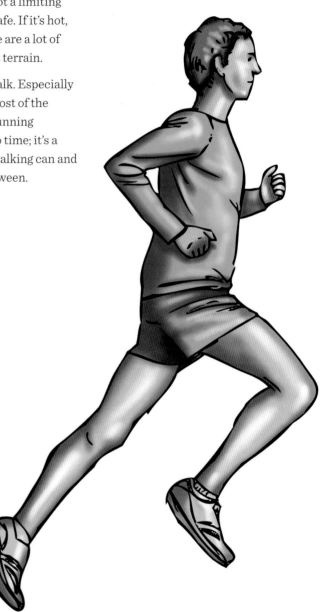

Form and Posture

Good posture (not hunching over, shoulders back, head up) while running helps your diaphragm expand fully and deliver the maximum amount of oxygen to your lungs. You should be leaning just slightly forward at the hips.

Try to run smoothly; don't bounce. When your body moves up and down, you're wasting energy. It's better to expend your energy to create forward motion rather than vertical motion.

Almost all your energy should be dedicated toward propelling yourself forward while running. Any muscles not being used for this effort should be as relaxed as possible. Don't flex your arm muscles. Have a comfortable bend in the elbow (around 90 degrees). Your hands should not be up by your chest or dangling low. Keep that bend as your arms move back and forth. Move your arms straight forward and backward while they're pumping, not across your body. Keep your hands relatively loose.

Remember to keep your face and breathing relaxed. Wincing or grimacing will not add anything to your forward motion. During most non-speed workouts, your breathing should not be too labored. You don't need to talk, but you should have enough oxygen to speak to someone comfortably.

Cadence

Cadence refers to your steps per minute. A higher cadence means higher efficiency. Nobody runs a race of any distance with long jump strides or baby steps. The perfect cadence is somewhere in between. If your cadence strides are quicker and shorter, your muscles delay fatigue and your breathing flows more smoothly.

A faster cadence means your feet touch the ground more times per minute. The time spent in the air isn't making you go faster at all. With each push off from the ground, you're propelling yourself forward. Keep your leg turnover high, and you'll stay efficient.

Hitting the Ground

When most people begin running, they land on their heel, roll their foot toward the front, and then push off with their toes. Others strike with their mid-foot, roll forward a bit, and push off on their toes. Most elite athletes land on their forefoot and then push off almost immediately.

When you're just starting out, you shouldn't worry too much about what kind of foot strike you have. Just go with the flow and try to concentrate on the other checkpoints of your form. However, the more forward you can land on your foot, the less forward momentum you'll lose each step.

Heel striking is equivalent to putting on the brakes a little bit with each step. Think about a sprinter, or go out and do a little sprint yourself: when sprinting very fast, you're up on your toes, spending very little time per foot on the ground and keeping a high turnover. When you get to the end of the sprint and want to slow down, you lengthen your stride and reach with your heel for several steps until you stop. You don't keep up on your toes and try to slow down with that form.

If you are a heel striker and want to transition to a forefoot striker, take your time. There's a big difference between the two running styles, and making the transition will probably stress your feet and lower legs. If you go this route, try to run on soft surfaces and allow for ample recovery between runs. Additionally, work on increasing your cadence, as your stride will naturally shorten and probably bring your strike closer to the front of your foot.

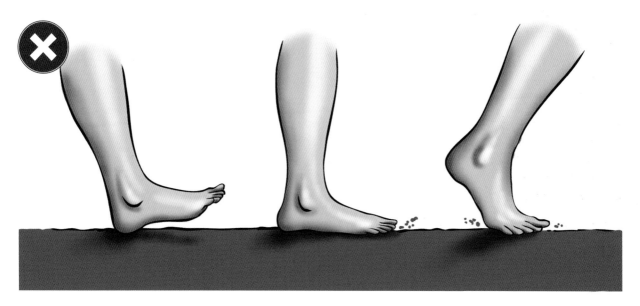

Heel striking can slow you down.

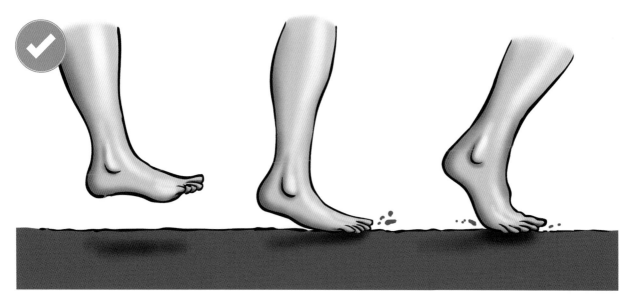

Striking with the forefoot is more efficient.

Fueling and Hydrating

In order to maximize your performance, your body needs proper nutrition and hydration before, during, and after long runs. Although it may feel awkward at first to carry nutrition on a run, it's essential if you're going to be out for over an hour, especially in hot and humid conditions.

Before Running

There aren't hard and fast fueling rules to follow, because what works for one person won't necessarily work for another. Experiment with various pre-run meals and different fueling options during your training. Before a morning run, oatmeal, bananas, or a bagel with peanut butter are all good choices. Mid-day, any normal lunch meal can work, but you'll want to avoid fatty foods and grease. Some triathletes choose to eat an energy gel or bar before a run. Try to give yourself between 20 and 30 minutes after eating before you head out for your workout.

In the weeks before your race, you'll have plenty of opportunities to try many different ways to fuel. Keeping track of how your body reacts to each helps you plan your nutrition in the future.

While Running

If you're out on a short training run or in a sprint-distance TRI, you might not need to replenish your calories before you finish. However, if you're out on a longer run (an hour or more), you'll need to fuel up during the run. It's difficult for most people to eat during the run, so you'll really need to learn what works for you.

As with biking, beyond "real food," your options will consist of products made with sugars, salt, and caffeine. During the run you'll burn calories and lose electrolytes; fuel will get you back in balance.

While it is easy to carry fuel while biking, running is a bit more challenging. You'll either have to hold it in your hand, use a pocket, or wear a fuel belt. If using a fuel belt, make sure to apply an anti-chaffing product to the area where it will rest. Even the best fitting belts will bounce somewhat.

Because of the portability question, nutrition is not the only important concern for fueling on the run. Keep in mind:

- Powder added to your sports drink or water to give you extra calories will not add additional weight, if you already plan to carry a water bottle.
- Energy gels are malleable and easy to swallow on the move. They are usually small enough to fit in the "key" pocket of your running shorts.
- Chewy gummies, jelly beans, or energy bars could make breathing more difficult because they require chewing.

If there will be aid stations in your race, try to find out what sort of nutrition they will offer. Training runs are a great time to become accustomed to the fuel you'll be offered when it actually counts.

Try to eat before you become hungry during your run. This will be difficult at first, as you may not yet know how your body will respond. An easy way to make sure you're getting your nutrition is to plan to eat on a schedule (e.g., every 20 minutes, you'll eat half a gel). You can adjust the schedule and amount of fuel based on your previous results and the difficulty of your workout.

After Running

When you finish a run, you'll want to eat a recovery snack. Again, it can pretty much be anything that works for you, but you'll want to make sure it contains both carbohydrates and protein. Energy bars are a good manufactured option, but more natural foods like bananas with peanut butter or even chocolate milk will get the job done.

It's critical to make notes after a training session on your nutrition strategy. Tweak your diet, before, during, and after your workouts to hone in on the perfect combination that works for you. When you find what agrees with you, you'll be that much closer to getting to the finish line with a smile. Just like practicing a good overall diet, we recommend variety.

On Race Day

Depending on the length of your race, there may or may not be aid stations. For shorter races, you'll need to supply fuel yourself. You may not need to fuel while running, but may eat a gel in the transition area after completing the bike. However, even if you don't need to fuel, you may have grown accustomed to running with a gel in your hand. During the race, continue to perform as you have in training.

For longer races, aid stations will be peppered throughout the course. Take in some fuel when it is offered, but always listen to your body.

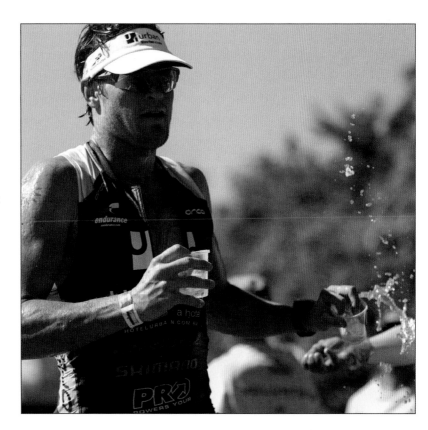

Outdoor Training

You can run just about anywhere, as long as you feel safe and you're able to find your way around. If you're aiming for an exact distance, map your run ahead of time or use a smartphone app or GPS watch to keep track of your mileage.

When to Run

Whenever possible, run during daylight hours. Running in the dark is dangerous because you are at risk of twisting an ankle or not being seen by a motorist. If darkness will set in before your run is finished, run with flashing red running lights (found at any sports store) attached to your front and back to make you more visible to others.

If you must run in the dark because of time constraints or other reasons, you need to be able to clearly see your path. Some companies have developed flashlights specifically for runners that illuminate both the path in front you as well as the ground at your feet. These devices cannot illuminate the path as well as daylight, but they're much better than running in the dark.

Keep an eye on the forecast when you are planning out your runs. Training in adverse weather will prepare you for anything, but it's best to plan around the weather when possible. Keep an eye on the forecast and try to plan your longer workouts for times when the weather will cooperate. During summer heat, try to get your runs done in the early morning or early evening.

Where to Run

Running gives a perfect excuse to get outside, breathe fresh air, and soak in the sunshine. There's never a shortage of places you can go run. Roads, sidewalks, trails, and forest preserves all over the country await you. Your path ahead may be concrete, asphalt, crushed limestone, dirt, grass, or any other surface. The softer the surface, the less impact on your body, specifically your feet, knees, and back. The harder the surface, the faster you'll go. We definitely recommend trading in some speed for less impact on your joints when you can. Also keep traffic in mind; the fewer cars there are, the safer you'll be, plus the air you breathe will be cleaner.

If you have the opportunity, give trail running a try. Trail running is highly recommended because of its lower impact and because of its uneven footing. It sounds counterintuitive, but studies have found that because trails aren't completely level, your legs actually get a benefit from running on these terrains. The little uneven surfaces of the trail help build up the small stabilizer muscles in your feet and ankles.

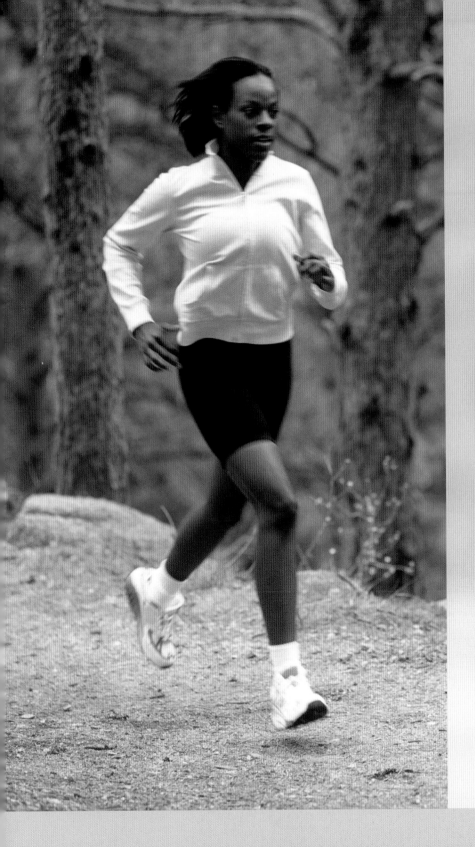

Trail Running Tips

- As always, run with a buddy whenever possible.

- Bring everything you might need, as there may be no water or bathroom breaks on the trail.

- Be sure your shoes have some support. No racing flats!

- Map out your route beforehand and keep track of where you're going.

- Check ahead of time for any sort of warnings in the area (flash floods, wild animals, etc.).

- If you can't find trails in your area, you can emulate trails by running on grass or dirt that runs parallel to a sidewalk or road.

Indoor Training

Even if you love nature, it's okay to train indoors sometimes. When the temperature reaches extremes or darkness falls, training outdoors can be dangerous. If the temperature is too hot, too cold, or too wet, it is best to find an indoor alternative for your workout.

Treadmills fit the bill when inclement weather or darkness sets in. They're also the perfect fit for people with bad knees or those who are carrying a few extra pounds. A treadmill's running surface is softer than any type of natural ground and absorbs much of the impact from running.

Consistency

Treadmills are great for teaching pacing consistency. If you set the machine to give you a 30-minute workout at 10 minutes per mile, you'll run exactly 10-minute miles. This great strength can also be a great weakness: your body may become conditioned to always expect a specific speed and surface grade. Your triathlon course will never involve a perfectly flat, entirely straight, weather-less run. If you do prefer running on treadmills, be sure you still incorporate several outdoor runs into your schedule before the big day. You don't want get into the run portion of a triathlon and be surprised that wind and hills actually do make a difference in your running! At a minimum, you should run with a 1-percent incline.

Speed and Incline

Be aware that treadmills can vary greatly from brand to brand. Some have variable inclines and several "programs" you can utilize to simulate a hill workout or a speed workout. The key factor is that you learn how to use the machine before you're in the middle of a workout. Locate the emergency stop button before turning anything on.

Also be sure you understand how to vary the speed and incline of the treadmill before starting a workout. If you do a hill workout, be aware that although the incline of the treadmill base increases, the speed most likely stays the same. If you're running outside and you hit a hill, your speed will naturally decrease. A treadmill doesn't account for this, so be prepared for your heart rate to go up for those intervals.

When on a treadmill, try not to always run at the same pace and incline. Even if your particular model does not have the ability to set specific programs, manually adjust your speed and incline from time to time during your runs, to force your body to adapt to changing conditions.

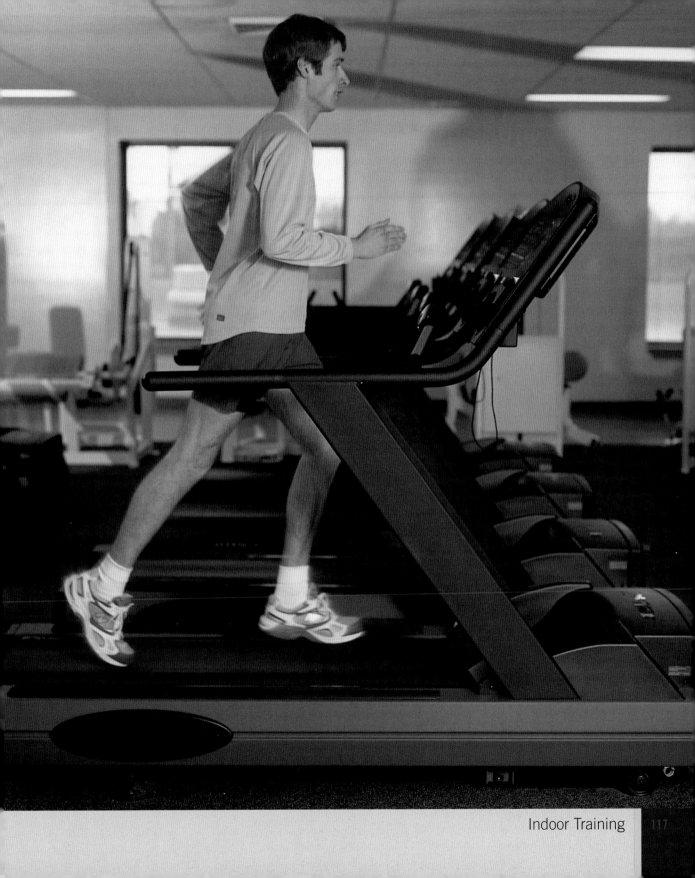

Running on a Track

If you feel more comfortable running on an outdoor track, go for it! Tracks usually are made of materials softer than concrete, and that helps keep the impact on your body low. Some people like tracks because they can be sure of the exact distance they run during a workout.

The downfall of tracks is the constant turning. On a quarter-mile track, a 3-mile run includes 1.5 miles of soft turns. Because our legs are designed to run in a straight line, turning this much in one direction can be harmful. One way to minimize the negative impact of turning (or at least share the impact between both sides of the legs) is to reverse directions at regular intervals. Switching directions every lap would balance your legs the most evenly, but would constantly interrupt your flow. Try reversing your direction every two laps, or even every mile.

If you can, stay away from indoor tracks or other tracks that are very short. These tracks force runners to go around 10 or more times just to run a single mile, and the angles can put too much stress on joints, muscles, tendons, and ligaments. Short tracks should be your very last option for workouts, and if used, should be done so very sparingly.

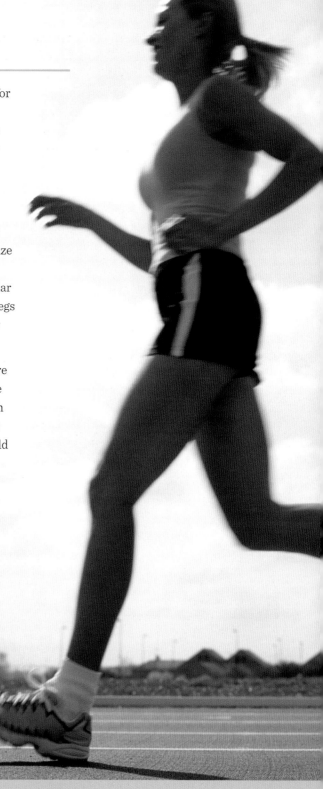

The Mental Game

In running, especially for people who are not elite athletes, the mental aspect is extremely important. We can't stress enough the importance of having a positive mental attitude as you're running. Where your mind leads, your body truly follows. Don't say to yourself, "I'm going to try to run four miles today." Instead, proclaim, "I am going to run four miles today." Believe in yourself. Believe you can do this. Remove all doubt, and if some tries to surface, just ask yourself, "Why can't I do this?" You'll find there's no reason.

Although some people are more naturally mentally tough, everyone can train himself or herself to be so. When people shift their attitude from I'll try to I will, it is amazing what will follow.

Think of it this way: you are a triathlete now. There is a workout plan in this book for you to follow. With each day, there is a fitness "recipe." You already have a daily routine: wake up, brush your teeth, eat breakfast, and go to work. Now you'll add: run four miles. Put it on your list and make it a priority, second only to family and work. If you decide that you're going to follow this recipe, and force yourself to mentally (or literally) put a checkmark next to each workout, you'll feel increasingly accomplished and motivated.

If you do find yourself in a poor mental state, remember that attitude is everything. If you're on the treadmill with nothing good to watch, you might want to invent a game of channel surfing—one channel per 60 seconds—you should be able to find a way to keep yourself entertained. Be creative and the minutes will tick by. Mental games work on trail runs just as well.

If you are someone who utilizes these mental games to keep your mind off the running, make sure to "check in with yourself" every once in a while to monitor your pace, breathing, and form. You will be successful!

Speed Workouts and Transition Runs

Once you've established a strong base by putting in several weeks of running, you can begin working on speed. Including speed workouts too early in a training program can overstress your body and possibly cause injury. Each speed workout is sandwiched between a warm-up to get the blood flowing before the session, and a cooldown afterward.

Speed work helps you live up to your fullest potential and also breaks up the monotony of your usual training runs. We highly recommend you try a few.

Fartlek

The best-named speed workout is the fartlek. Fartlek is Swedish for "speed play." A fartlek workout involves a warm-up and then a series of periods where you pick up speed. After each pick-up, you go back to the regular speed. After you've done your designated number of pick-ups, you can finish your run.

The pick-up during a fartlek is not a sprint. You don't want to push your body to the breaking point. You're simply picking up the pace for a bit and then going back to your normal speed. The period used can be marked by feel, distance, or time.

Tempo Runs

Tempo runs consist of a warm-up, an up-pace run, and a cooldown. The up-pace portion of this workout is not a sprint, but a bit of a pick-up from your normal pace. With this speed workout, you should calculate the full distance you'll run as precisely as possible, as well as at least four intermediate distances. This enables you to confirm that your pace is consistent throughout the run (for example, for a mile pick-up at a 10-minute-mile pace, each quarter mile should be 2 minutes, 30 seconds). You can measure exact distances using a smartphone app, GPS watch, or heart rate monitor with speed tracking. The first time you do this sort of workout, you might want to try just a half-mile tempo run. Start out slow and be sure you stay consistent; consistency trumps speed. Your warm-up and cooldown will be around 10 to 15 minutes each and should increase as the tempo run distance increases. A good rule of thumb is to keep the tempo run distance about the same distance as your warm-up distance.

Intervals

Intervals might leave a bad taste in your mouth if you ever had a track coach who pushed you to the limit. This workout involves a warm-up and then several "intervals" of fast-paced running over a specific distance/time, with plenty of rest in between. During the rest, an extremely slow jog is recommended, although walking is permitted at the start of the rest period. The interval distances/times can vary depending on the training plan you're going for.

Initially, most workouts are based on running for a specific amount of time. Distance is not nearly as important as the amount of time you put in. After you establish a base and are ready for some speed work, you'll start to incorporate fartleks, tempo runs, and intervals. A sample interval workout might include a 10- to 15-minute warm-up and then four faster 400-meter (or yard) intervals, each with about a minute rest in between. Follow the speed workout with a cooldown.

Transition Run

Transition runs (T-runs) are those you run within a few minutes after completing a bike workout. Don't get nervous about this, all you're doing is helping condition your body to do what it'll need to do in the race: transition from cycling to running. Your leg muscles need to get used to going from the circular pedal stroke to the rhythm and movement of running.

Work T-runs into your schedule whenever you can. Each week of training usually has one or two longer rides built into the schedule, and you'll see that almost all of them have a T-run immediately following to condition your body to go from one discipline to the next. Your muscles will feel strange when you get off the bike and start running; they have to get into a new groove. Practicing this often will make it that much easier on race day.

Preparing for a T-run helps you practice what to bring on the day of the race. There's no better way to find out that you forgot to include something vital than to do it during a training workout. Before leaving for your ride, lay out all the equipment and food you'll want to take on your T-run. These things shouldn't be different from what you bring on a normal run.

After your workout, make notes about how the transition went: what you did well and where you need to improve.

T-runs will seem awkward at first. Give it time, and they'll begin to feel normal. You'll do so many of these during training that it will be almost like second nature during a race. Keep in mind that unlike speed training, you don't need a base prior to initiating T-runs. These should begin early on in your training.

Drills and Accelerations

Drills and accelerations are two more ways to improve your speed. These two techniques are not exactly workouts; they're more like the icing on the cake at the end of a run session. You can take a short break after your workout, but it's best to do these while your muscles are still warm and loose. Both drills and accelerations help increase your foot turnover and, therefore, your speed. These are not difficult, but the payoff can be tremendous.

All you need to do drills and accelerations is a straight, flat area where you can run unimpeded for about 100 yards (or meters). Dirt trails or tracks work well, but flat grassy areas or bump-free sidewalks are fine, too. Just be sure to examine the area first so you aren't surprised by any uneven ground. You can choose to do each of your drills for a number of repetitions (20 each leg) or for a specific distance (from the edge of the sidewalk to that tree over there).

Butt Kicks

In this simple drill, you work on the part of your stride that's behind the midpoint of your body. You should already be warmed up from your main running workout. From your "starting line," you can take a couple steps to get moving. Then, while continuing to run, try to kick up one of your heels and hit your butt. Repeat with the other foot.

When this serious butt kicking is going on, your feet will be moving quickly off the ground but you won't be moving forward that quickly. That's fine. Don't worry if your heel isn't actually touching your butt in the kick. The important thing to improve your speed is to get the essence of the motion right.

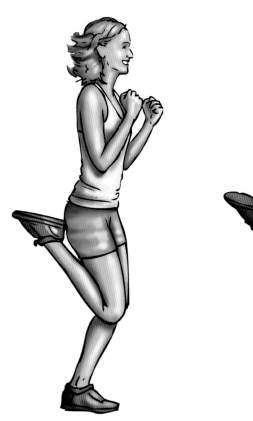
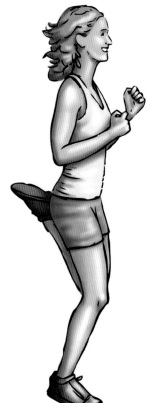

High Knees

High knees keep your feet moving at the same speed as butt kicks, but your focus shifts to keeping your legs in front of you (instead of behind you). Just take a couple steps and then start lifting those knees. You might feel like a soldier marching in double time, and you'll probably need to lean back a bit to balance yourself. Don't try to lift your knees so high that you risk pulling something, but do get them even with your waist (or higher) if you can. Keep yourself in control the entire time.

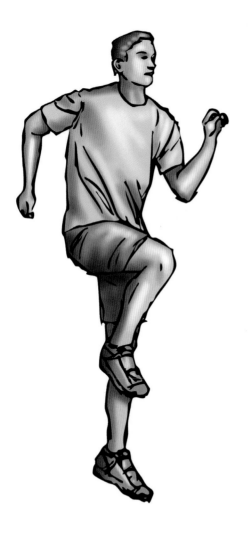
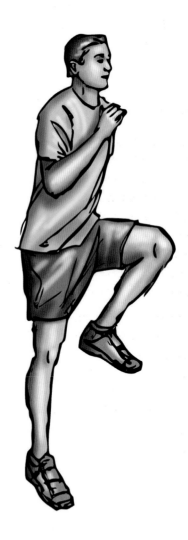

Side-Stepping Cross-Overs

This drill is a great way to get some of your leg stabilization muscles firing. The movement is similar to the sideways movements in some line dances except your foot speed is much faster.

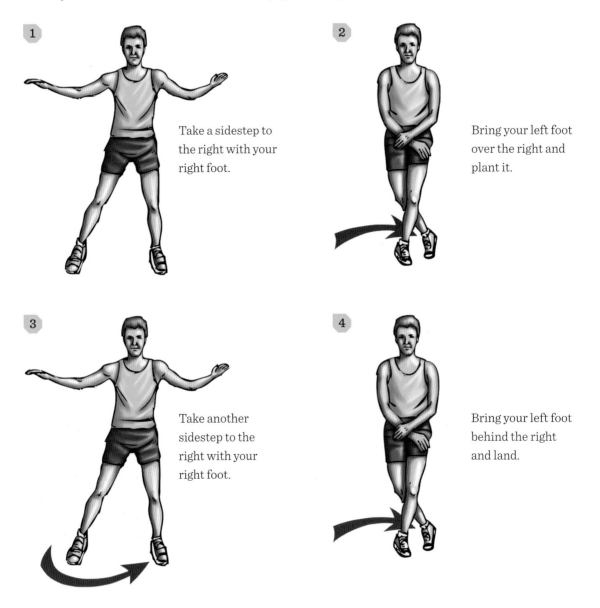

1

Take a sidestep to the right with your right foot.

2

Bring your left foot over the right and plant it.

3

Take another sidestep to the right with your right foot.

4

Bring your left foot behind the right and land.

Repeat steps 1 through 4 until you cover your goal distance or number of steps. Then head back to the left side doing the same thing.

Skipping

This time you're working on the front part of your stride. Even if you don't know how to skip in the traditional sense, the exaggerated movement we show you will teach you in no time. Again, you can begin from your "starting line" with a few steps of jogging. Then, whenever you decide, instead of putting your foot down immediately after bringing it forward in a stride, raise one of your knees as high as you can. At the same time, raise your opposite arm (same symmetry as when you're running normally). The momentum of your raising knee and your raising arm causes you to rise a bit off the ground with your back leg. Then, when your first leg comes down, repeat the same motion with the opposite leg. You're skipping just like a kid.

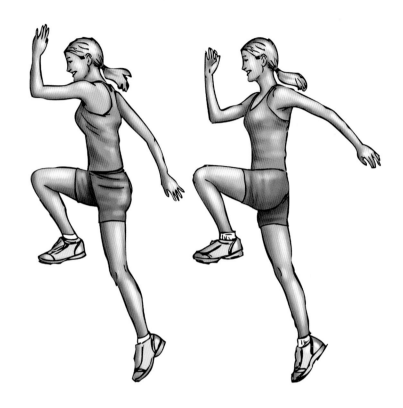

Accelerations

Accelerations are exactly what they sound like. Instead of running at a constant speed, you accelerate for a given distance (100 meters or less; about the distance of a football or soccer field). Don't worry if you think this sounds tough; we promise it isn't that bad. With this drill, you start off with a slower pace and then speed up a bit. Then after a few more steps, accelerate a bit more.

At no time should you be in an all-out sprint, but by the end, you should be running much faster than normal. When you hit the "finish line," slow down until you're either jogging or walking. Catch your breath for a bit at the finish line and then turn around and do another acceleration in the opposite direction. You could also jog or walk to the "starting line" as your breather and do your next acceleration in the same direction. Start off doing four of these after a workout and quickly build up to six.

With long, low-intensity runs, mixed in with speed workouts and drills, you'll see your improvement in your running in very short order.

Prepare for the Unexpected

A few unexpected things can happen when you're out running. As with everything in life, preparation is key.

Check the Weather

If you scout out the weather forecast in advance, you should be able to plan your run accordingly. If it starts to rain during your run, the most important thing to remember is that everyone's visibility will be worse (especially drivers on the road), and that the pavement or trail will become more slippery. Rain or shine, use extra caution with traffic on the road, as the drivers may be talking or texting and not even realize you are there.

Stay Hydrated

The best way to avoid problems with nutrition and hydration, is to always bring more of each than you think you will need. Whenever you go for a run, get in the habit of bringing at least one energy gel, even when you think you won't use it. If there is no water supply available, run with a bottle in hand. If you realize you are short on either hydration or nutrition, do not try to push yourself to some predetermined distance. It is best to turn around and start heading back. Once you're back at home base, fuel up and continue your run. If you are really in a bad place physically, don't be afraid to phone a friend to come pick you up.

Prepare for Injuries

Unfortunately, injuries are another "unexpected" that can come with running. If you are not accustomed to running, you may feel as though your body is falling apart after the first couple of runs. The key is to understand the difference between soreness and injury. Most people experience some soreness when they first start running. That soreness should go away as your muscles become accustomed to the program. If you have nagging pains that don't feel like regular soreness, get checked out immediately by your doctor. The fix might be as easy as putting orthotics in your shoes or working on some exercises to strengthen specific muscles.

If you do find out that you have an actual injury, take the necessary time to get yourself back to where you need to be. You absolutely cannot rush injury recovery; to do so is to set yourself up for re-injury or worsening of your condition. Be smart. If an injury keeps you from participating in your planned triathlon, you will be extremely frustrated. Instead of beating yourself up about it, keep in mind that there will never be a shortage of races. This experience will only make you a better triathlete in the long run.

If a shoelace breaks while out on a run, you might need to get creative. If it breaks near one of the ends, you should be able to inch it through the eyelets in one direction to give yourself enough lace at each end to make a bow or knot. If it breaks at a less convenient spot, you may need to work with what you have and create two mini-laces, using part of the lace to tighten the bottom eyelets and part of the lace to tighten the top eyelets.

Safety Check

The best way to stay safe while running is to use common sense.

Run Against Traffic

Per pedestrian rules, if you have to run on a street, run against traffic. That way, you can keep your eye on the vehicles coming at you instead of turning your back on them. This doesn't significantly decrease closure time between you and any cars, but it does give you great visibility as to what is coming your way. If you live in a place where cars drive on the right, stay as far left as possible, on a shoulder or on the sidewalk.

Carry Pepper Spray

It may seem like overkill, but pepper spray is easy to carry and can save your life if used correctly. You'll be able to find it in most specialty stores. This doesn't just apply to women; anyone running alone is vulnerable. Pepper spray provides a convenient and effective means of defense, including against aggressive dogs.

Run with a Buddy

Whenever possible, train with a buddy. It will add camaraderie, encouragement, and safety to your workout. The buddy system is always encouraged in all forms of exercise, from swimming to weight lifting, and running is no different. However, we know that it's not always possible to find a running partner who shares your exact same fitness schedule or level. Try to work out with a buddy whenever you can, but if that's not possible, or you feel like working out on your own, go for it. Just use your head. Have your phone and pepper spray handy, and be sure someone knows where you're headed and when you'll be back.

Safety Checklist

- ◊ Take pepper spray if you're running alone.
- ◊ Always bring a cell phone and some emergency cash.
- ◊ Know (at least generally) where you're headed.
- ◊ Know how to get back to where you started.
- ◊ Bring hydration and nutrition with you.

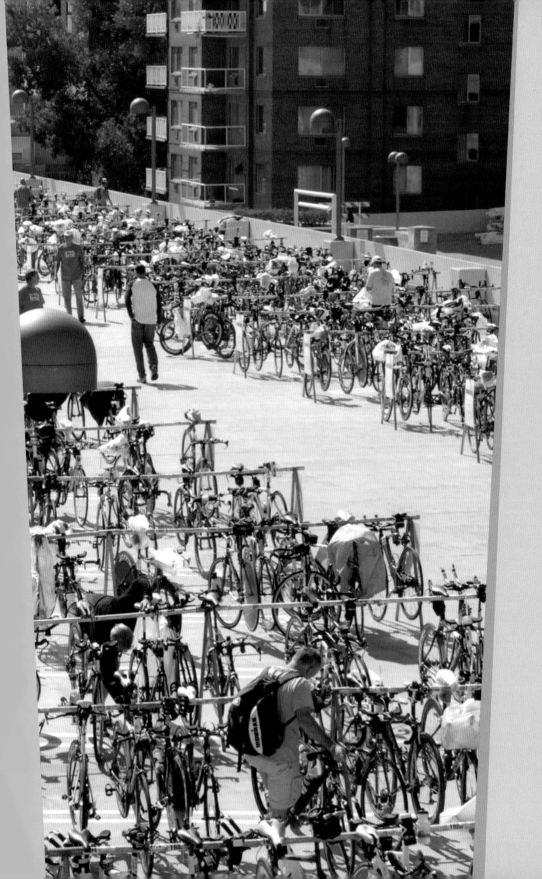

Transition

Transition is one of the hardest parts of triathlon for beginners to grasp. Your race consists of three disciplines—swim, bike, and run. Between each discipline, you have a few minutes to change equipment, muscle groups, and mind-set. This is the transition. Changing equipment during all the excitement can be a little rough. Using different muscle groups and adopting a new perspective while starting the bike or run can be even more challenging.

This part covers techniques and strategies for practicing transitions in your regular workouts, so when race day comes, you'll be ready.

PART 6

Transition Basics

The transitions in a triathlon are numbered by sequence. Your first transition, or T1, is between the swim and the bike. Your second transition, or T2, is between the bike and the run.

The concept of a transition is easy:

1. Find your gear within the transition area.

2. Drop off the equipment you no longer need.

3. Pick up the equipment you need for the next segment.

The key is to bring everything you need or think you might need. It's better to be over-prepared with some extra items than to find yourself missing something.

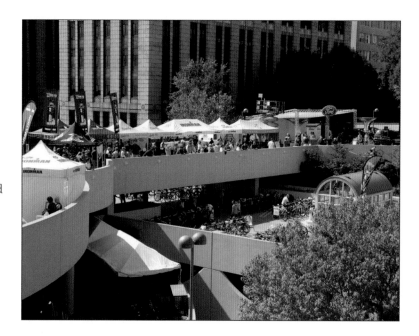

The Transition Area

The transition area is almost always the same location for T1 and T2. This space is filled with rows of bike racks that look a little like elongated metal sawhorses.

Each row is usually numbered with ranges based on the race numbers of participants. Your designated transition spot will be where your race number is. If there is no designation, then you'll stake your claim on a spot you can remember. Your transition space may only be as large as a beach towel. It is small, and you are packed in with the other triathletes. Clearly label your gear and keep it on your towel.

Transition areas are usually in a wide open space, like a field or parking lot, where hundreds of bikes and gear will fit. Race organizers always try to put the transition area close to the water to limit the distance that the triathletes need to run upon finishing the swim.

For shorter races, you will check in and set up your transition area the day of the race. For longer races, you will check in and set up transitions the day before the race. Bikes and extra gear are left in the area in either case, and the honor system is in full force as security is typically limited.

Setting Up for Transition

A smooth transition requires thoughtful planning. Lay out all the gear you'll need for the upcoming sport in your designated spot. When you come in from the previous event and complete your transition, the spot for your upcoming sport should be void of gear. That's a great way to be sure you have everything.

By nature of the pace of a race, you're going to put some pressure on yourself during your transitions. Keep your wits about you. To avoid making mistakes, keep things as simple as possible and set up your transition area in a way that forces you to go step-by-step through the gear you need to switch out.

Group all your equipment by sport, and then place the equipment for each sport in order, with the things you will put on or use first closest to where you will be standing or sitting. The stuff for use last goes furthest away on the transition towel.

If you really want to know exactly where each piece of equipment will go before you get to your race, divide up a towel into sections using a magic marker. Label each section with the item it will hold and then you won't have to worry about equipment positioning on race day.

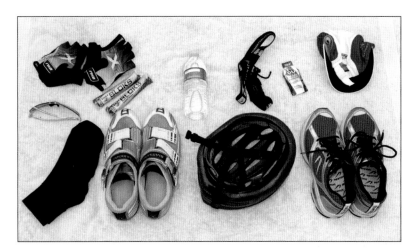

Practicing Transitions During Workouts

Set up your practice workout transition area just like you would in a race. When planning for a transition workout, prepare ahead of time. You don't want to waste time organizing between events.

When you've decided what items you'll need and what you'll be wearing for each segment, you then have to figure out where and how you're going to perform the transition. Depending on your training location, you might choose to set up your T-gear at home, in the trunk of your car, or in a gym locker.

Through practice and perseverance, you'll figure out how best to set up your transition area and go through the steps to be successful. Have fun with all the planning, practice, and strategy involved.

Transition 1: Swim to Bike

How do you feel after a swim workout? You're probably wet, thirsty, and maybe hungry. Maybe you also need to use the bathroom. Those are the four main things to mark off the list during T1.

Drying Off

During a race, many choose to air dry to avoid spending time toweling off. During a swim-to-bike transition workout, you might decide you want to dry yourself a bit before heading out on the bike leg. If so, have a towel (other than the one your gear is set up on) handy in your transition area.

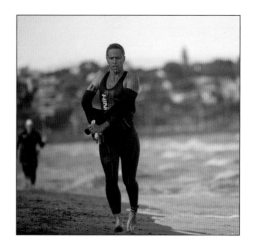

Changing Clothes

Depending on the length of your race, designated changing areas may or may not be available. While many people choose to change during practice workouts, few people do so in shorter races, which typically won't have designated changing areas. We recommend only changing clothes if the designated changing areas are available. If you're uncomfortable being out of the water in just a swimsuit, you can always slip some shorts or a shirt on over the suit.

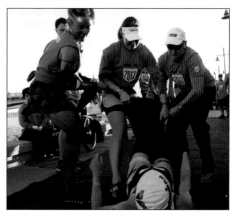

If you are in a longer race that allows wetsuits, there may be "wetsuit strippers" waiting for you at the exit of the swim. These generous race volunteers will literally help "strip" you out of your wetsuit by pulling on the sleeves and the legs of the suit. Once stripped, they will hand you your wetsuit to carry on to T1.

Gathering Your Gear

You should have everything you need for the bike portion of the race laid out on your towel and ready to go. You'll need the same things you've used during training: a helmet, sunglasses, jersey, shorts, and shoes. Do you also use socks or bike gloves? What about some sort of body lubrication? Nutritional items and supplements? Water bottle(s) or sports drinks should be on everyone's list.

Fueling and Hydrating

Many people find it difficult to eat anything right after the swim, but if you're able to, take a few bites of your nutrition of choice. At the very least, have water or a sports drink at the ready in your transition area and pack some additional nutrition for your ride.

Timing

The time it takes to complete T1 will depend upon many factors. The transition clock starts after you complete your swim. Some triathletes spend as little as 60 seconds in transition while others may take 5 to 10 minutes. There is no exact target to aim for as it varies depending on the course layout, race distance, and weather. Try to move as quickly as you can, but don't rush.

When setting up your practice T1 (or T2), you might decide to put your hydration bottles in a fridge or cooler to keep them cool. If you do, be sure to put a big sign on your bike reminding you to get them out and on your bike before heading off.

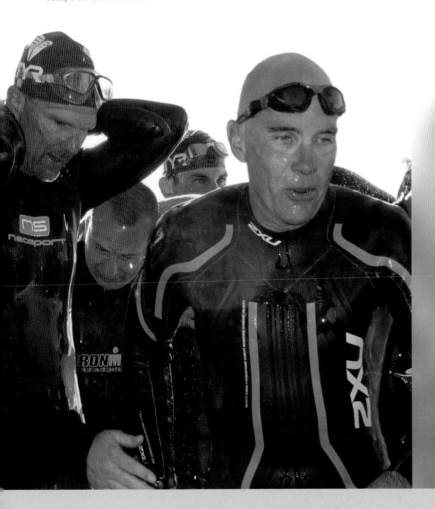

T1 Step by Step

Take off wetsuit (if applicable).

Drop your goggles, swim cap, and wetsuit in your T1 area.

Reapply sunscreen.

Rinse your feet with bottle of water.

Change into biking clothes if needed.

Put on socks.

Put on your race number (on a race belt or pinned to your jersey).

Eat and drink as needed.

Use the bathroom if necessary.

Put on helmet, sunglasses, and bike shoes.

Pack nutrition as needed.

Walk your bike to the mounting zone.

Transition 1: Swim to Bike

Transition 2: Bike to Run

T2, your second transition, is more straightforward than T1 because you have fewer things to pick up on your way out. You drop off a lot of gear, but have little that you need to put on before you start the run.

Think about how you feel after a long bike ride. Are your legs tired? Water bottles empty? Are you hungry? Make mental notes during training (and actual notes after the workouts) that will help you tailor your personal transition lists.

Think about your essentials for running and have these ready to go for T2. You'll need sunglasses, a jersey top, shorts, and shoes. Do you use a hat or a visor? What about socks? Do you usually lube up in certain areas? Be sure to pack all these things you'll use.

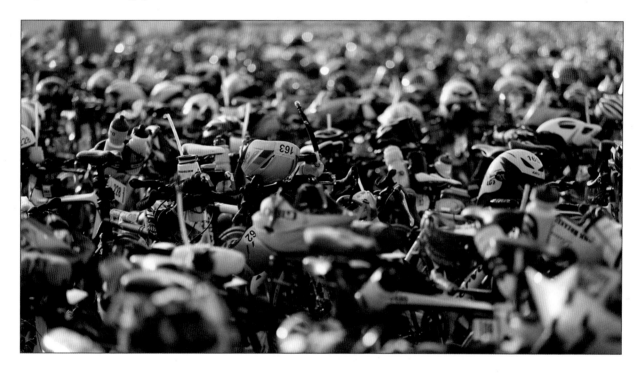

Some people elect to change clothes between the bike and run segment. This is rare in a race that's shorter than a half-Ironman, but it can be done. Just follow the steps in the T1 transition. Many people choose to change before a T-run while training because they're not being timed, and comfort outweighs speed. If you're comfortable running in bike shorts, keep them on and save yourself a little time.

If your bike has clipless pedals or you have specific shoes for the bike, you'll need to change into running shoes during T2. If you bike with your running shoes, you're good to go; no change is necessary in that department.

T2 Step by Step

Rack your bike.

Take off your helmet and bike shoes and place in your area.

Change clothes if needed (transfer your bib to the new jersey if not using a race belt).

If using a race belt, rotate your race number to the front.

Reapply sunscreen.

Eat and drink as needed.

Use the bathroom if necessary.

Put on your running shoes and running hat.

Put on your running belt and hydration system.

Pack nutrition as needed.

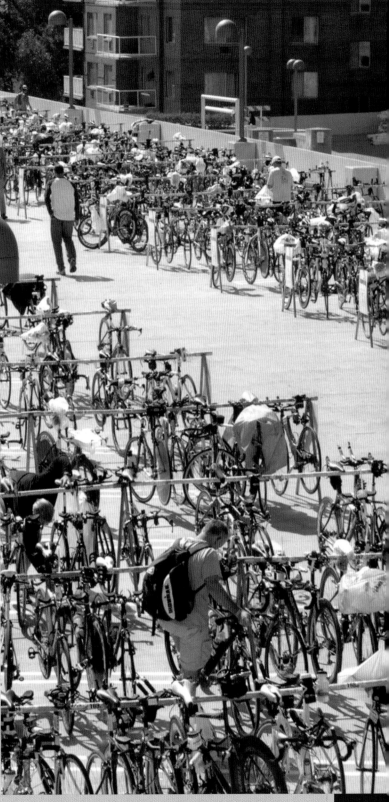

Race Day Transitions

When race day comes, you'll be prepared from all your practice. Believe in your preparation. Utilize your checklists. Bring anything you might want or need.

Packing Your T-Bag

One of the major differences between T-workouts and actual races is that you need to transport all your gear and your bike to the race site. Backpacks, duffle bags, or specialized TRI bags are usually the tool of choice. Whatever method you use, be sure you also practice packing up all your gear a couple days before the race. This helps avoid a late-night scramble the day before the race.

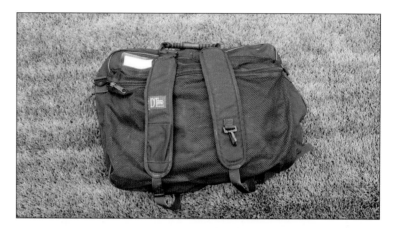

On race day, remember that you won't arrive, set up, and start racing immediately (unlike training). Be sure to bring any little extras you'd like to have with you, and lay them out on the transition towel separate from everything else. That way, they'll be at your disposal when you're setting up your T-area, and you'll be able to grab them on your way out. Extra food or drink, warm clothes, and things to keep you entertained fall into this category.

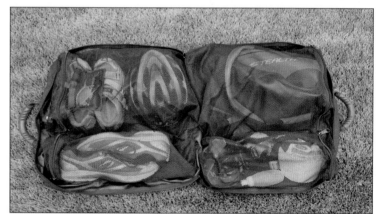

What About Valuables?

There aren't usually special gear checks for valuables like phones, keys, and wallets. If you choose to bring valuables, have a plan to manage them before the race begins. Typically, race venues allow for spectators to stand just outside the transition area where you can hand off your valuables to a friend or family member, which is the best option. However, if you happen to be doing a race without your own spectators, leave your phone and wallet in your car, and do your best to hide your keys in your gear in the transition area, like in a rolled up towel or shoe. Triathletes trust the honor system in transition.

For Longer Races: Special Needs Bags (SNBs)

At Ironman races, there's one spot on the bike course and one spot on the run course where you can pick up a bag of goodies that you have packed in advance. These two special needs bags (one for the bike, one for the run) are simple plastic drawstring bags that will be given to you when you receive your race packet. Before the race, you fill the bags with items you'd like to have during the bike and run. Generally, triathletes fill the bags with items that aren't available from the course aid stations and include anything from first aid items like antibacterial ointment, to functional items like another water bottle, to favorite treats like candy bars or cookies.

Your SNBs are identified with your race number or name, so volunteers can easily get them to you. You pack the two bags at your leisure and turn them in at a special location the morning of the race. The race volunteers then take them to the midpoint (or near it) of the bike and run courses where you'll pick them up later in the day.

When receiving your SNB, race volunteers will try to get you the bag quickly, without you having to slow down on the bike or run. If you have to wait, keep in mind they are doing the best they can. Once you have your SNB in hand, you can slow down to grab what you want and drop what you don't. Some efficient triathletes can grab their bag and continue without slowing their pace, but that can be very difficult. Especially if it's your first time, don't rush yourself. Get everything arranged exactly like you want it before getting back into race mode.

Depending on the race, you might not get your SNBs back. Don't put anything in a SNB that you absolutely want to have after the race is done. Pack your bag with items you might want during the race but you won't miss if you never see them again.

Transition Checklist

To help you keep track of what you need (and don't need), here's a sample transition checklist.

General

- ❑ Contact solution
- ❑ Eye drops
- ❑ Transition hydration
- ❑ Transition snack
- ❑ Change of clothes
- ❑ Post-workout nutrition
- ❑ Sunscreen
- ❑ Keys
- ❑ Phone
- ❑ Cash
- ❑ First-aid kit with bandages, cortisone cream, over-the-counter painkillers, medication for indigestion, and hydrogen peroxide or rubbing alcohol

After Swimming

- ❑ Towel
- ❑ Bottle of water to rinse off your feet

For Biking

- ❑ Bicycle
- ❑ Helmet
- ❑ Bike shorts
- ❑ Jersey or singlet
- ❑ Bike shoes
- ❑ Socks
- ❑ Lubrication
- ❑ Sunglasses
- ❑ Frame-mounted pump, CO_2, spare tube(s), and bike multi-tool
- ❑ Floor pump
- ❑ Water bottles and energy drinks
- ❑ Nutrition for bike segment
- ❑ Heart rate monitor

For Running

- ❑ Shoes
- ❑ Socks
- ❑ Shorts
- ❑ Jersey or singlet
- ❑ Sunglasses
- ❑ Hat
- ❑ Fuel belt
- ❑ Nutrition for run
- ❑ Hydration for run
- ❑ Lubrication and liquid bandages

Logistics

Distance and weather are the biggest influencers of what you decide to wear for each leg of the race. A complete change of clothing at each transition is not typical, but as with most things in triathlon, your comfort is what matters the most. Some of these items are optional, and you should adjust the list based on your personal experiences and preferences.

Remove everything you no longer need after coming in from one leg, and then put on everything you need for the next. Take a breath, get a drink, grab something to eat, and do a quick inventory so you have everything you need before you head out again.

Timing

If you are new to triathlon, plan to take your time in transition, both in workouts and in races. It won't take long for you to cut time and eliminate steps from your transitions, but don't rush. During workouts, try to begin your second event of a transition workout within 10 minutes of finishing the first event, but if it takes a little longer to get going, don't beat yourself up over it. Taking your time only adds a minute or two, whereas rushing can ruin your time in the next event.

Prepare for the Unexpected

If you've never participated in a triathlon before, a lot of what you encounter may be "unexpected." If you have the opportunity, go watch a triathlon in person. Sit by the border of the transition area for a while and watch the triathletes going through T1 or T2. This is the best way to learn what to expect.

If you're not able to visit a triathlon in person before your race, talk to experienced triathletes, especially those who have completed the course you plan to run. Every race transition area has similar aspects, but there will always be nuances to setup, location, and flow that make each race unique.

Protection from Weather

Transition areas for shorter races like sprints or Olympic distances are bare bones; they are almost always outside and usually do not offer any cover from the elements. You are switching gear and changing clothes in the same space where you just racked your bike. There are no fans or showers, no spritzers to cool down or heaters to warm up. At half and full Ironman races, bikes are always outside on a rack, but sometimes there are inside areas in a building or large tent for changing, warming up, or cooling down. Again, there are no standards or rules to transition setup. Do your research and be prepared.

Bathroom Breaks

In every race, there are portable bathrooms in or near transition areas. You may have to wait in line, but it's better to use them if you need to. Do not plan to use the portable bathrooms to change clothes.

Missing Gear

When you pick up your gear after the race, review your transition checklists as your inventory guide. While extremely rare, if you find that you are missing any gear, check the lost and found first, and if necessary, contact the race authorities for the proper procedures to follow up on the claim.

Safety Check

The most important safety recommendation during transition is to be aware of your surroundings. Triathletes will be running around in all directions with their minds focused internally. Do your best to keep from bumping into each other in what can be frantic minutes of quick changes.

Entry and Exit

Bike and run traffic in and out of the transition area is monitored and directed by race authorities or volunteers. In T1, those coming in from the swim leg and those going out on the bike leg will not collide, nor will the bikes collide with the runners going out on the third leg of the race. While there are no absolutes, there are usually designated "entry" and "exit" areas at either end of the transition space to keep traffic smooth.

In every race, regardless of distance, you will always walk or jog your bike when you are in transition. In T1, your helmet must be clipped before exiting the transition area, and you will be penalized or disqualified from the race if you ride your bike before the designated line is crossed. Coming into T2, you must get off your bike before the designated line and walk or jog your bike back to your transition space.

Physical Issues

If your body is giving signs that something is wrong, listen. Transition is a good time to regroup and make sure you have a good read on your health. Are you overheated, too cold, or losing energy due to lack of nutrition?

You might have developed a blister on the previous leg of the race; dry your skin and apply a bandage from your first aid kit. Do you notice chaffing in one area of your body? Apply some lubrication. Is your stomach churning? Grab the appropriate nutrition or medical remedy.

Make sure you address warning signs. If there is a health concern, let someone know. That way you can get the medical attention you need. This is true in transition as well as at any point in the race.

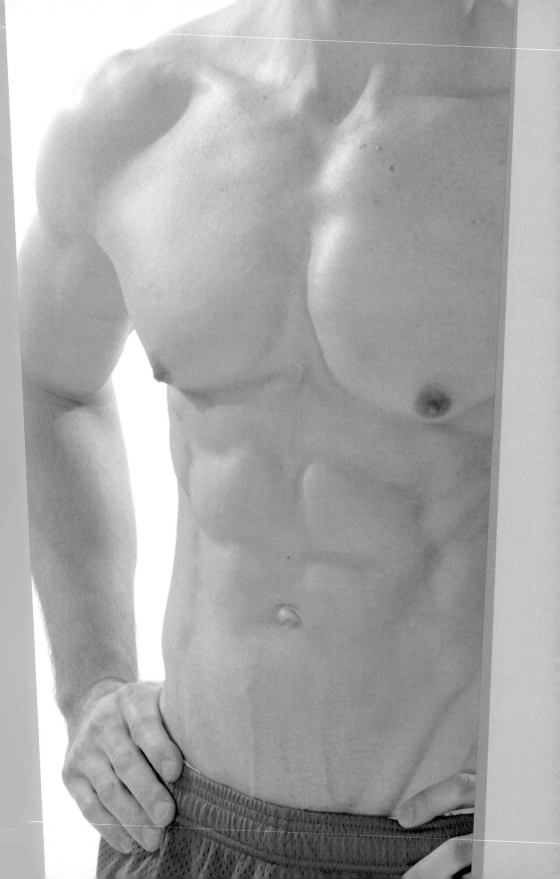

Strength Training and Stretching

Strength training and stretching play an important role in your conditioning program for a triathlon. Consistent strength training and stretching will both improve your overall experience and reduce your chance of injury. This part includes 40 exercises that you can incorporate into your training schedule to build strength and flexibility.

Strength Training

The reason to incorporate strength training into your triathlon training regimen is simple and obvious: it makes you stronger. The stronger and more conditioned you are, the better you'll be able to adapt to and progress in the sport of TRI. Strength training also improves *time to exhaustion,* or the level at which you fatigue, which helps prevent injuries. This is critical to TRI, especially as the distances increase.

The 26 strength training exercises in this book were chosen based on sport specificity, muscle groups, and planes of motion, with a focus on functional training. Some of the exercises only require your own body weight, while others require gear such as dumbbells or exercise bands.

We recommend you perform 8 to 12 exercises, 8 to 12 reps of each exercise, for 1 or 2 sets, 2 or 3 times a week, alternating upper body and lower body exercises. This is an ideal way to maximize and balance endurance with recovery.

Feel free to go directly from a shorter cardio workout into your strength training. If you need to break it up into two sessions, just make sure to warm up the muscles before the strength training begins.

Warm-Up

As with any workout, the first step in a strength session is the warm-up. You can warm up with a low-level aerobic activity like walking or cycling, or you can begin the workout with a set of exercises using lighter weights. The objective is to gradually increase your heart rate, blood pressure, oxygen consumption, and muscle elasticity. Skipping this step could lead to injury.

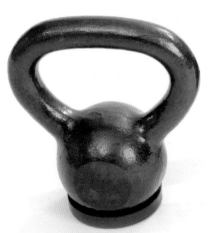

Main Workout

The main workout session consists of repetitions (*reps*) and *sets*. Reps are the number of times you do a specific exercise or movement, and a set refers to the total number of reps as a whole. For example, 3 sets of 10 means you would perform 10 reps of an exercise for 3 rounds. Completing the reps and sets of multiple exercises represents completing a *circuit*.

The *load* (resistance utilized) depends on where you are in the program. We recommend starting out gradually to allow your body a chance to condition itself. Keep the weight light and the number of reps on the higher end of the 8 to 12 range. The best way to determine the right amount of weight to use (when applicable), is by trial and error. You should be able to do 8 to 12 reps with good form. Although this is the normal range for most exercises, some core exercises vary up or down, and in these cases, it's best to go by feel—your muscles should feel worked, but not exhausted.

There are two phases within the movement: the work, or shortening (*concentric*) and the return to its resting state, or lengthening (*eccentric*). For example, in a bicep curl, the concentric phase occurs when you lift up the weight; the eccentric phase occurs as you lower it. Many people think only about the work portion of a movement. However, the lengthening component is just as important. The recommended tempo is 1 or 2 seconds concentric and 2 to 4 seconds eccentric. Some exercises may incorporate longer holds, such as the plank, which you might hold for 20 seconds or more.

Opinions differ on how much *rest* you should take between sets. Some say rest as you need it, with less at the beginning and more toward the end of a workout. Others say to rest 30 to 120 seconds between sets for a moderate strength training program. See what feels right for you. The amount of rest you require between sets depends not only on where you are in your workout, but also on how much weight you're lifting.

Cooldown

As with your hard aerobic sessions, each lifting session should include a cooldown. You can do the same activities as you did for your warm-up or try something else. Just slow things down for 10 minutes or so. The objective is to gradually lower your heart rate and blood pressure and to process post-exercise hormones and lactic acid.

Strength Training Workouts

The goal in TRI strength training varies depending on what part of the program you're in. Generally speaking, the goal is to increase strength in the off-season and earlier in your racing program. As you get closer to your race, the focus shifts from strength building to maintenance.

By focusing on strength training 2 or 3 times a week and alternating between upper and lower body exercises, you'll maintain intensity by resting some areas while working others; this results in an efficient workout session. If possible, try not to lift weights two days in a row as your muscles need time to recover and rebuild.

The following pages include instructions for 26 different strength training exercises. When choosing which exercises to do, incorporate variety based upon the equipment you have, the areas on which you need to focus, and the balance between upper, lower, and core movements.

To help you with your selection, we have grouped the exercises based on muscle focus and their main foundational movement; some of them appear in more than one group. Choose at least one exercise from each group as you build your circuit. This will ensure you have a well-balanced program.

As you get started, here are some general guidelines to follow:

- Start gradually; ease into your training.
- Use controlled movements, and always have control of the load.
- Use a full range of motion for optimal gains.
- Incorporate variety—mix up the order, change loads.
- Maintain good posture and body alignment in all movements.

Listen to your body during your workout, especially in the beginning. It knows how far it can go and when you've pushed too far. *This is hard,* is an okay thought to have while working out; however, *this is painful* is not.

Group 1: Planking
Plank

Suspended Band Side Plank

Kettlebell High Plank Row

Bridge

Medicine Ball Push-Up

Group 2: Pushing
Suspended Band Chest Press

Medicine Ball Push-Up

Dumbbell Shoulder Press

Bench Dip

Group 3: Pulling
Dumbbell Pull Over

Dumbbell Bicep Hammer Curl

Kettlebell High Plank Row

Group 4: Lunging
Medicine Ball Lunge with Twist

Dumbbell Lunge

Lateral Lunge

Group 5: Rotating
Wood Chopper

Medicine Ball Lunge with Twist

Group 6: Hinging
Dumbbell Straight-Leg Deadlift

Kettlebell Swing

Suspended Band Hamstring Roll

Medicine Ball Slam

Group 7: Squatting
Dumbbell Squat

Suspended Band Squat and Single Leg Squat

Other Exercises
Dumbbell Lateral Raise

Standing Calf Raise

Stability Ball Crunch

Stability Ball Back Extension

Safety Check

Prior to attempting any of these programs, get approval from your doctor. Once you begin strength training, pay attention to your form and be sure to perform all the exercises with proper technique.

Strength and flexibility training is an ideal way to augment TRI conditioning. It challenges your body in ways that the three sports of TRI alone cannot. The results and benefits are many, and not just in the short-term. These principles can help improve your physical quality of life in the future as well. Balancing strength training, flexibility, and TRI-specific conditioning is the best way to reach your full active lifestyle potential.

Plank

The plank is a foundational movement that sets the stage for many other exercises. When performed properly, the plank engages your core as well as upper-body stabilizing muscles.

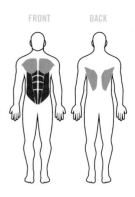

FRONT   BACK

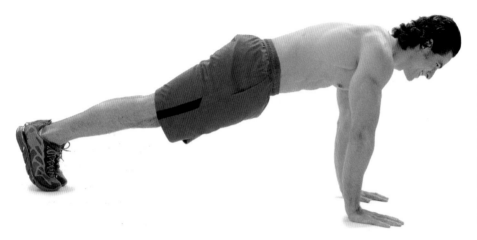

Get into a push-up position on the floor. Hold yourself up off the floor keeping your shoulders, hips, knees, and ankles in alignment. Take deep breaths while contracting your abs to keep your body up in the plank.

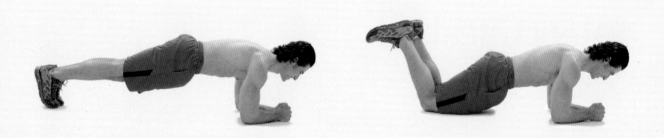

You can also get into the plank position from your forearms, keeping your abs contracted and your shoulders over your elbows. If you feel pressure in your lower back, drop your knees down to the floor.

Suspended Band Side Plank

Planking with suspended bands adds challenge and a level of instability to the traditional side plank. You must control your feet and the other gravitational forces in play.

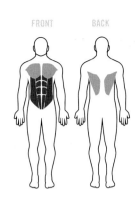

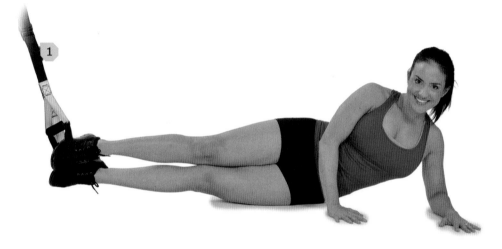

Lie on your side with your feet in the bottom straps (foot cradles) of the suspension bands and one forearm resting on the floor.

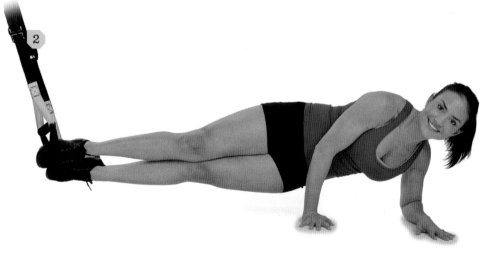

Lift your hips up to create a straight line plank with your body. Breathe deeply while holding the plank. The free arm can support you for balance on the floor, rest on your side, or be lifted up toward the sky.

Kettlebell High Plank Row

This exercise takes the plank and adds in a row that works you head to toe with a focus on the core and back muscles—the rhomboids and lats. If you don't have a kettlebell, you can use a dumbbell instead.

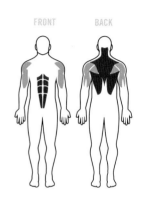

FRONT BACK

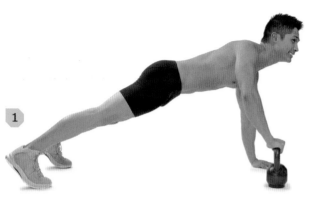

1 Hold yourself up in a plank position with one hand on the floor and the other holding the kettlebell.

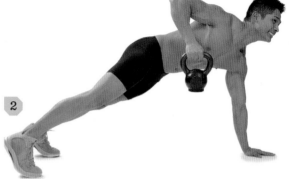

2 Inhale as you pull the kettlebell up to your side. At the top of the row, your elbow should be at a 90-degree angle.

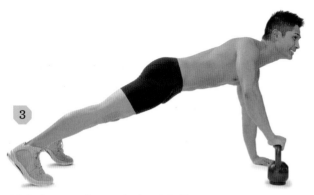

3 Exhale as you lower the kettlebell to the floor, then transfer it to the other side and repeat.

> If you have difficulty staying in plank position, perform this exercise from your knees.

Bridge

This is a great exercise for the core, glutes, and hamstrings. For an added challenge, perform this exercise with your feet on a step, bench, or stability ball.

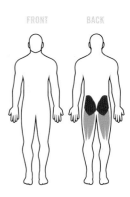

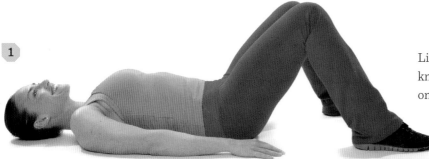

1 Lie on your back and allow your knees to bend. Keep your feet flat on the floor.

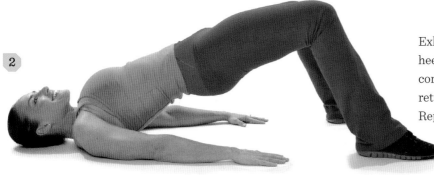

2 Exhale as you press though your heels up into the bridge. Keep your core engaged. Pause at the top and return to the starting position. Repeat.

Stability Ball Crunch

This exercise works your core and lower back by challenging your balance throughout the movement.

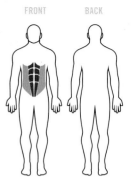

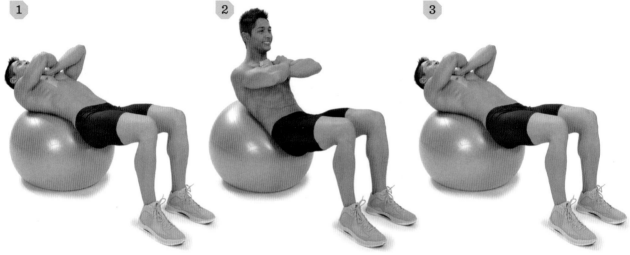

1 Lie on the ball with your arms crossed and your head and shoulders slightly lifted. Inhale as you stretch your abs.

2 Exhale as you lift your shoulders and contract your abs at the top of the crunch. The ball should stay in place.

3 Inhale as you return to the starting position. Repeat.

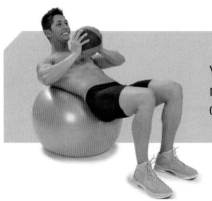

You may choose to hold a medicine ball or weight at your chest for an added challenge.

Wood Chopper

This dynamic move can be done with a medicine ball, kettlebell, or other free weight. The rotation in the torso works your obliques.

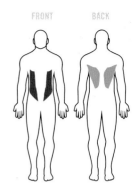

FRONT   BACK

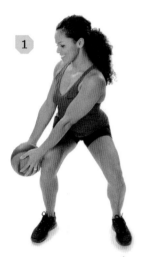

1 Hold a weight down at one side of your body. Stand with your feet shoulder width apart, facing forward, in a half squat.

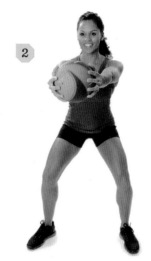

2 Inhale as you swing the weight up to one side of your body, stretching your abs and obliques.

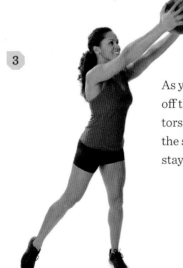

3 As your back heel comes off the floor, allow your torso to twist slightly to the side while your hips stay facing forward.

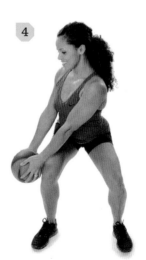

4 Exhale as you chop down toward the opposite knee, returning to the starting position.

Medicine Ball Lunge and Twist

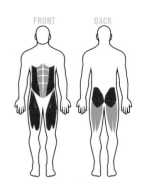

This exercise targets your quads, glutes, and hamstrings as you lunge. Your core stays engaged as you work to maintain balance with the weighted twist.

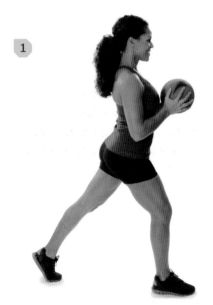

1

Stand with one foot in front of the other, with equal weight between them, and bring your back heel off the ground. Hold the medicine ball at your chest with both hands.

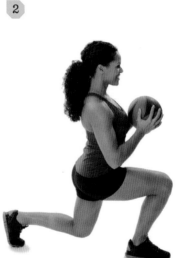

2

Inhale as you lower into the lunge, creating a 90-degree angle with your knees.

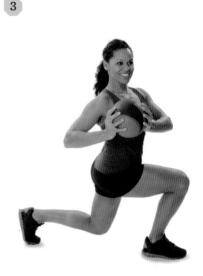

3

Exhale as you contract your abs and twist toward the front leg. Drive the move from your torso and allow your head to move with your shoulders. Inhale as you ascend back to the starting position.

Repeat as desired, then switch your leg position and work on the other side.

Suspended Band Hamstring Roll

This exercise engages the core and targets your glutes and hamstrings. The instability from the bands adds challenge and requires balance.

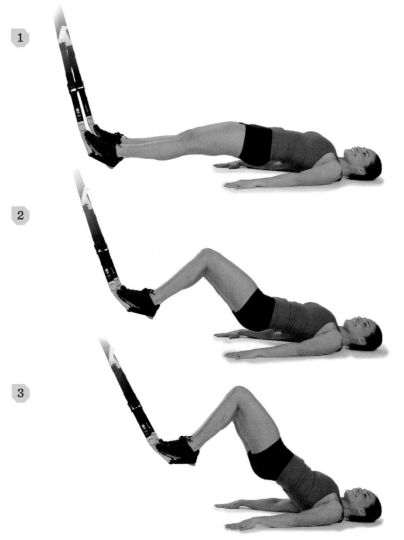

1

Lie on your back and place your heels in the suspension bands (foot cradles). Lift your hips and lower back off the floor, creating a straight line with your body.

2

Exhale as you pull your feet in to contract your hamstrings.

3

At the top of the roll, your knees, hips, and shoulders should be in a straight line. Inhale as you roll your heels back out to straight legs and return to starting position.

Suspended Band Chest Press

To perform this full-body move properly, you must engage your core and use stabilizing muscles for control.

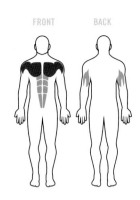

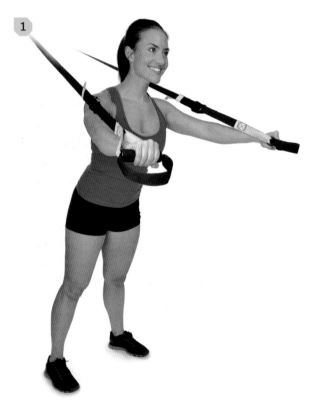

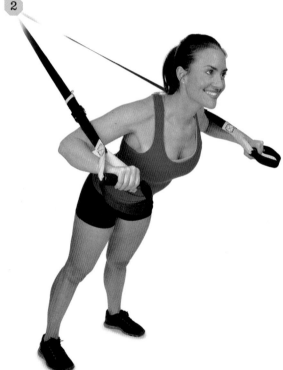

Holding onto the handles with your palms facing down, lean away from the anchor point of the suspension bands.

Inhale as you lower your body, creating a 90-degree angle with your elbows. If the band rubs your arms, lift your hands slightly. Exhale as you ascend back to starting position.

Kettlebell Swing

This dynamic exercise demands power from your hips, core, glutes, and hamstrings as you swing the kettlebell into the air.

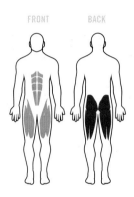

FRONT   BACK

1

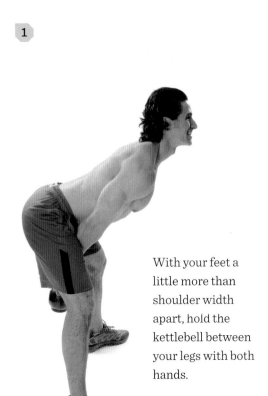

With your feet a little more than shoulder width apart, hold the kettlebell between your legs with both hands.

2

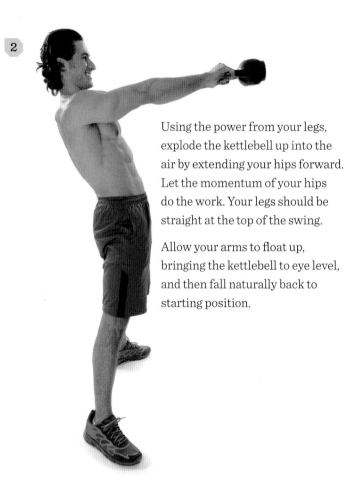

Using the power from your legs, explode the kettlebell up into the air by extending your hips forward. Let the momentum of your hips do the work. Your legs should be straight at the top of the swing.

Allow your arms to float up, bringing the kettlebell to eye level, and then fall naturally back to starting position.

Bench Dip

The bench dip opens up and stretches your shoulders while targeting the arms and triceps.

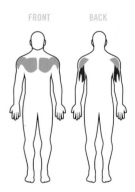

FRONT   BACK

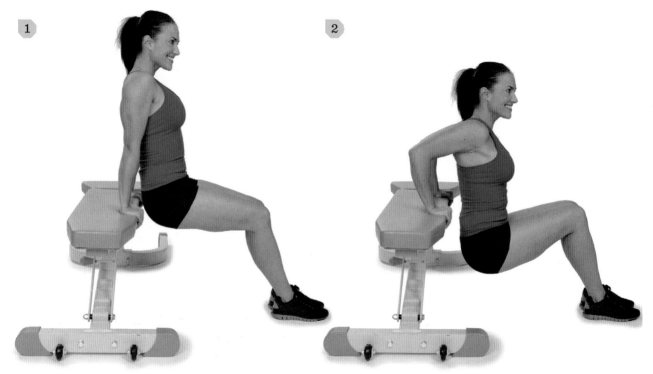

Place your hands behind you to hold you up, letting your hips hang off the bench. Your feet should be out in front of you on the floor.

Inhale as you lower your body by bending at the elbows.

At the bottom of the dip, your elbows should be at a 90-degree angle.

Exhale as you push your body back up to starting position. Maintain good posture and keep your body near the bench.

Dumbbell Lunge

Lunges are another foundational movement that build lower body strength and coordination. The dumbbells allow you to add load after you have mastered the movement.

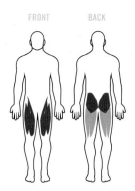

FRONT   BACK

1

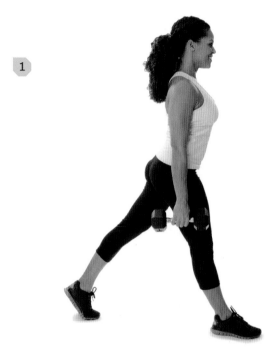

2

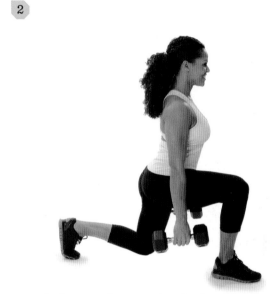

Holding your dumbbells at your sides with arms straight, stand with one foot in front of the other, and distribute your weight equally between them.

Allow your back heel to lift as you maintain good posture and inhale and lower into the lunge.

Pause before your knee reaches the floor. Your legs should be at approximate 90-degree angles. Be careful not to extend the front knee past your toes.

Press through your heels and exhale as you rise back to the starting position.

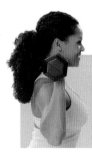

To incorporate more core engagement, hold the dumbbells up to your shoulders.

Medicine Ball Slam

This functional exercise is a powerful move that works the entire body and has a cardiovascular conditioning effect.

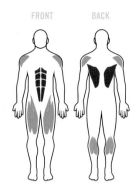
FRONT   BACK

1

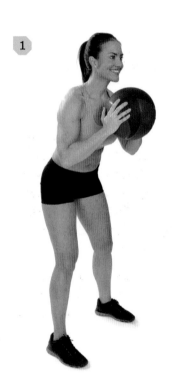

Stand with feet shoulder width apart. Hold the medicine ball at your chest.

2

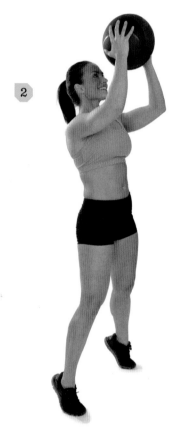

Inhale as you stretch your abs by lifting the medicine ball above your head.

3

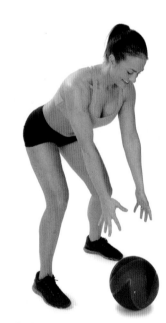

Exhale as you contract your abs and bring your torso forward to slam the medicine ball down in front of you. Allow your head to travel with your shoulders.

Some medicine balls bounce, others do not. If the ball bounces high enough, catch it as you squat and return to starting position. If it doesn't, squat down, pick it up, and return to starting position.

Dumbbell Shoulder Press

This exercise works your shoulders and upper back, while standing adds to the functional training aspect.

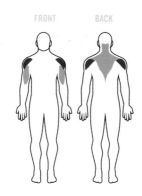

1

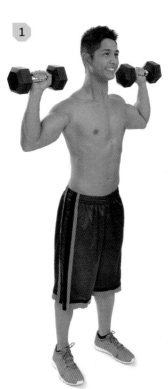

Stand with your feet shoulder width apart. Hold the dumbbells up at your shoulders.

2

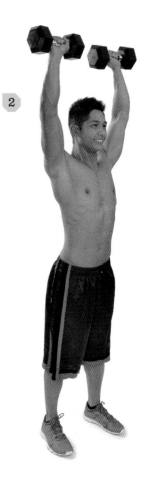

Exhale as you raise the dumbbells straight up. Keep your core engaged while maintaining good posture. At the top of the press, straighten your arms.

Inhale as you control the dumbbells back to starting position. Repeat.

Dumbbell Straight-Leg Deadlift

This move targets the major muscle groups of your lower body, including your glutes, hamstrings, and quads.

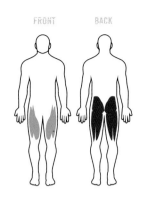

1

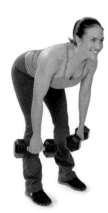

Stand with feet shoulder width apart and a slight bend in your knees. The dumbbells should hang comfortably in your hands in front of you.

2

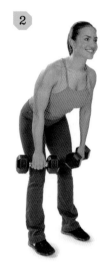

Bend at the hips to stretch your hamstrings. Make sure you have a soft bend in your knees and keep your back flat.

3

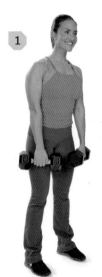

Keep your shoulders down and back as you rock your hips back for a slight pelvic and hip tilt. Inhale as you lower the dumbbells. Keep your weight in your heels.

4

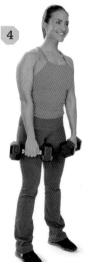

Exhale as you ascend and pull the dumbbells back up to starting position.

Dumbbell Squat

This exercise builds on the bodyweight squat by adding load with the dumbbells. It targets the lower body and core.

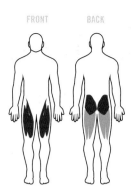

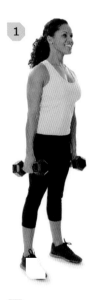

1

Holding your dumbbells at your sides, stand with your feet shoulder width apart. Keep your bodyweight in your heels.

2

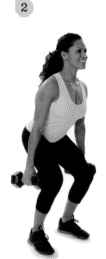

Shift your hips back to create a natural arch in your back. Inhale and squat down, keeping your chest up.

3

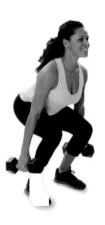

At the bottom of the squat, your legs should be at approximately a 90-degree angle. Make sure your knees do not go over your toes.

4

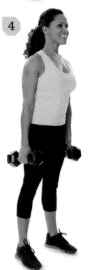

Exhale as you rise back to starting position while maintaining good posture.

Suspended Band Squat

Using the suspension band allows you to focus on proper form by off-loading some weight through your arms. This exercise targets your glutes, hamstrings, and quads.

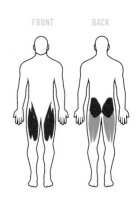

FRONT   BACK

1

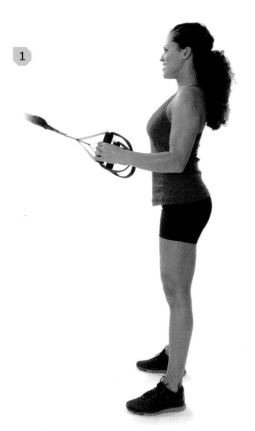

2

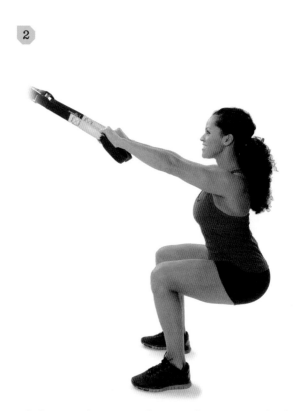

Stand with your feet shoulder width apart. Hold the handles of the suspension bands in your hands, arms bent at approximately 90-degrees, and lean back.

Inhale as you lower into the squat, keeping your back flat and your abs engaged. Create a 90-degree angle with your knees. Exhale as you rise back to starting position.

Use your arms to help control balance and assist with the movement as necessary.

Single Leg Squat

Once you master good form with both legs in the suspended band squat, you can try the single leg version. Again, this exercise targets your glutes, hamstrings, and quads.

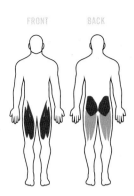

FRONT   BACK

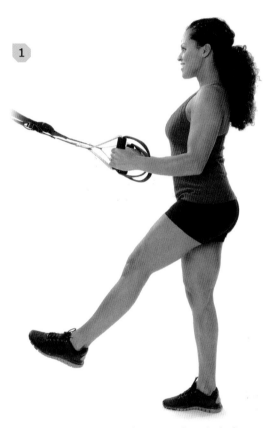

1

With suspension bands in your hands, balance on one leg with your opposite leg extended. Lean back into a sitting position with the extended leg out.

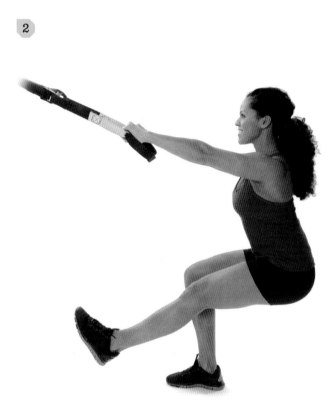

2

Inhale as you lower into the squat, creating a 90-degree angle with your knee. Exhale as you rise and return to starting position.

Two-Hands-On Medicine Ball Push-Up

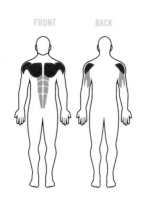

FRONT   BACK

Unlike regular push-ups, push-ups from a medicine ball require both strength and balance. The medicine ball creates instability, requiring the stabilizing muscles in your upper body to engage. Both the one-handed and two-handed versions of this exercise target your pecs, delts, triceps, and core.

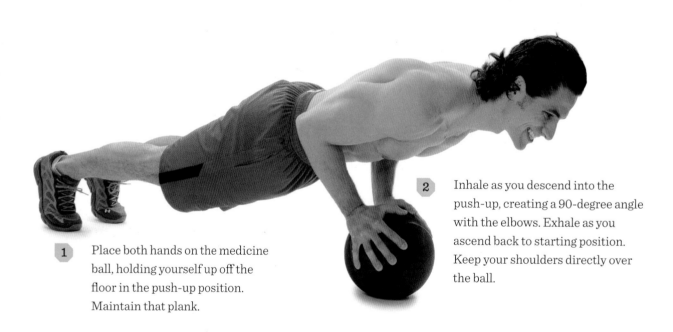

2 Inhale as you descend into the push-up, creating a 90-degree angle with the elbows. Exhale as you ascend back to starting position. Keep your shoulders directly over the ball.

1 Place both hands on the medicine ball, holding yourself up off the floor in the push-up position. Maintain that plank.

One-Hand-On Medicine Ball Push-Up

Once you mastered the two-handed medicine ball push-up, try performing the movement with just one hand on the ball.

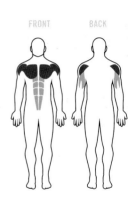

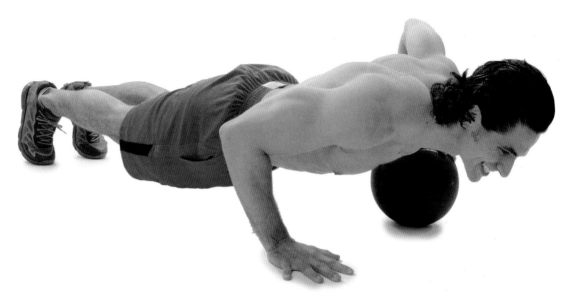

1. Place one hand on the medicine ball and the other hand flat on the floor to hold yourself up in the push-up position.

2. Inhale as you descend into the push-up, creating a 90-degree angle in the elbows. Exhale as you ascend back to starting position.

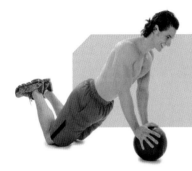

If your lower back becomes stressed or if you have difficulty maintaining proper form, perform the movement from your knees.

Dumbbell Lateral Raise

The lateral raise with dumbbells targets your shoulders, specifically the medial deltoids (middle of shoulders). This is a good exercise to build strength for swimming.

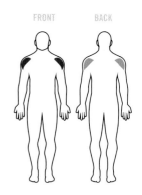

FRONT   BACK

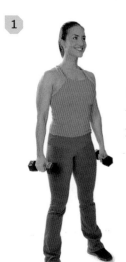

1

Stand comfortably with the dumbbells down at your sides.

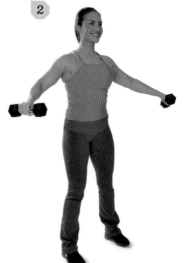

2

Exhale as you lift the dumbbells out to your sides. Your shoulders should be relaxed and your arms slightly bent.

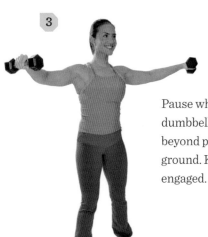

3

Pause when the dumbbells are just beyond parallel to the ground. Keep your core engaged.

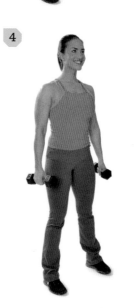

4

Inhale as you control the weights to the starting position.

Dumbbell Pullover

This exercise effectively works many muscles in the upper body, with the lats and chest as the primary drivers.

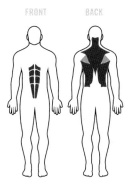

FRONT   BACK

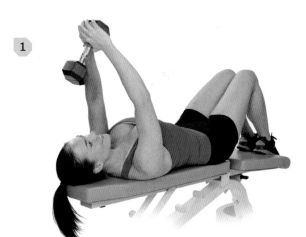

1 Lie flat on a bench with your arms stretched straight up. Hold the dumbbell vertically at one end of the weight.

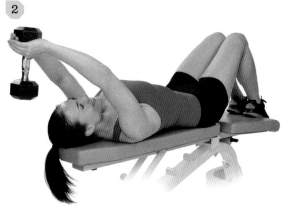

2 Inhale as you lower the dumbbell behind your head.

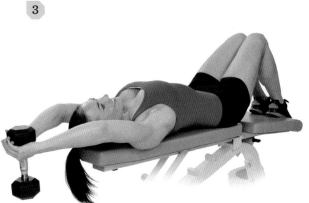

3 Pause and stretch your back and abs out once you have fully lowered the dumbbell. Engage the core with a slight bend in the elbows.

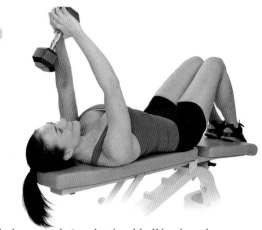

4 Exhale as you bring the dumbbell back to the center of your body.

Stability Ball Back Extension

This exercise targets your core and lower back with a reverse crunch on the stability ball.

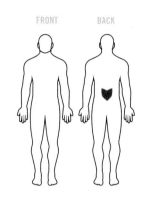

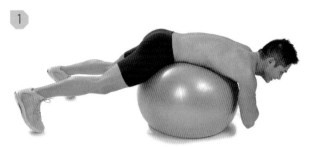

1. Lie over a stability ball on your stomach, with your arms crossed in front of you and your feet on the floor for balance. Inhale as you engage your abs. Your feet will help keep you stable.

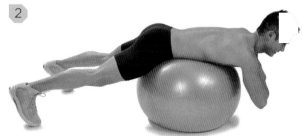

2. Exhale as you bring your torso up to contract your lower back.

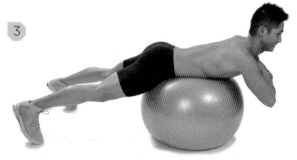

3. Extend up until your shoulders, hips, and knees make a straight line.

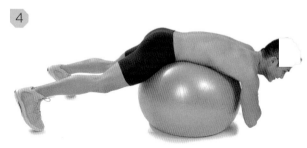

4. Inhale as you return to starting position.

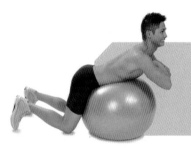

If you need more stability, rest your knees on the floor. Also make sure you're using an appropriately sized ball for your body.

Dumbbell Bicep Hammer Curl

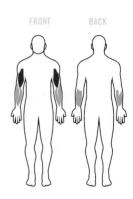

FRONT   BACK

The hammer curl uses a neutral grip (palms facing in) that closely resembles your hand position on the bike. This change in grip targets your biceps and forearms.

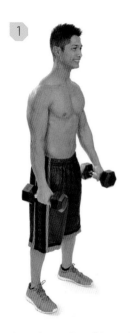

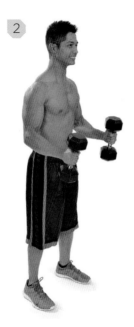

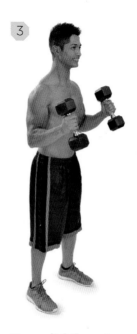

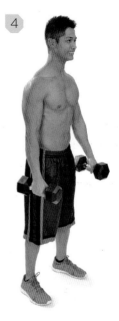

1 Stand comfortably with the dumbbells down to your sides and your palms in a neutral grip. Keep your shoulders back and relaxed.

2 Exhale as you hinge at the elbow to curl the dumbbells up.

3 Pause slightly past 90-degrees and squeeze your biceps. Keep your elbows near your sides.

4 Inhale as you lower the dumbbells back to starting position.

Lateral Lunge

Lunging to the side mixes things up by moving in a different direction. It's important to train in various angles and planes of motion to challenge and recruit different muscles. This approach provides greater muscle symmetry, dynamic balance, and reduces chance of injury.

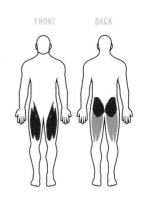

FRONT   BACK

1

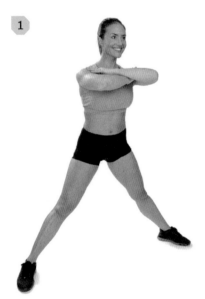

Stand with your feet outside of your shoulders for a strong, wide stance. Keep your back straight and lean slightly forward.

2

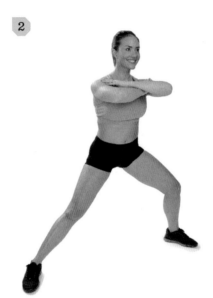

Move your hips back for a slight pelvic and hip tilt. One leg should be straight while your other leg performs the entire lunging movement. Keep your weight in your heels.

3

Inhale as your lunging leg lowers down to one side. Exhale as you ascend back to starting position.

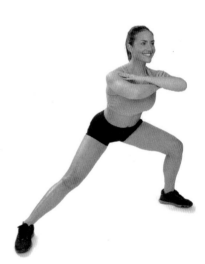

Holding a weight or medicine ball at chest level while performing this move will add an extra challenge.

Standing Calf Raise

Working your calves with this exercise will both strengthen and help stretch your lower legs.

FRONT   BACK

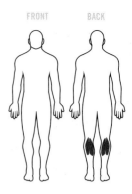

 1

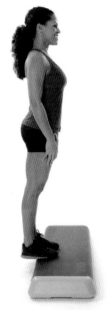

Position the balls of your feet on the edge of a step. Hold on to a bar or wall for support if needed.

 2

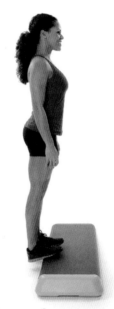

Inhale as you lower your heels below your toes to stretch your calves.

3

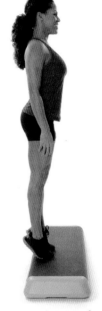

Exhale as you raise your heels up past your toes. Squeeze your calves tight at the top of your extension. Inhale as you descend back to starting position.

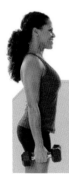

For an increased challenge, hold a weight or weights by your side.

Stretching and Flexibility Training

Stretching makes you flexible, and good flexibility is critical for increased performance, reduced injury, better recovery, improved muscular balance, and postural awareness. When you exert force to lengthen muscles and tendons at the right intensities, in appropriate durations, and with some frequency, you increase connective tissue flexibility. This book includes stretches that cover all areas of the body, with special attention to the muscles used during triathlon training.

When to Stretch

The best time to stretch is when your muscles are warm, right after your workout session. Studies suggest that stretching when your body's tissue temperature is slightly elevated produces a greater permanent (plastic) deformation. Performing the same steps with a cooler tissue temperature only produces temporary tissue elongation. After a workout session, cool down and flow right into your stretching routine while your body temperature is still elevated and your muscles are supple.

As with strength training, there are many schools of thought regarding stretching. Some believe you should only have a focused session two to three times a week. Others say you should stretch every day. We recommend stretching after all workouts whenever possible; even if you only get in one quick set for each major muscle group. Spending a few minutes stretching can save you hours and even days in recovery and prevent injury.

Some opt to designate a day or two every week to spend more time stretching. Consider adding more sets and duration to each stretch. For example, if you perform 1 set at 30 seconds duration of each stretch post workout, you could add 2 or 3 more sets at 60 seconds duration on these designated days. If you're going to stretch at a time not directly following a workout, perform a 5 to 10-minute warm-up first.

How to Stretch

Three popular types of stretching techniques are:

- Static

- Dynamic

- Proprioceptive neuromuscular facilitation (PNF)

Static stretching is the most widely accepted method of stretching. It involves a slow, gradual, low-intensity stretch. The intensity is the point at which you begin to feel a slight discomfort, but not pain. Generally, you would hold a stretch for 10 to 30 seconds, and repeat each stretch 2 to 4 times.

Dynamic stretching is an active stretch done through a full range of motion. It is done in a slow and controlled manner. The theory behind it is to mimic activities that are dynamic (such as a golf swing).

PNF is composed of many strategies. One of the more commonly used aspects of it deals with a contract-relax sequence. Essentially, you would flex (contract) with maximum force or strength at the end point of a limb's range of motion. This is an isometric movement. You hold it for approximately 5 to 10 seconds and then relax and apply an easy stretch.

Although all three methods have their benefits, we recommend using the static stretching technique with the exercises in this book.

Maintaining Flexibility

Degree of flexibility decreases with age. As people get older, there's a shift in collagen fibers and in overall hydration in and around soft tissue structures. If you're under age 30, you probably won't need to hold your stretches as long as someone who is over 30 years old. After the age of 30, you need to start increasing the time you hold your stretches (up to 60 seconds) to receive the same benefits.

When stretching, it's important to remember the following:

- Low-intensity, long-duration stretching is most conducive for lasting benefits.
- Warming your tissue temperature prior to stretching contributes to increased range of motion and lasting benefits.
- Target specific joints and muscle groups when you stretch, and maintain that specific focus.
- Hold most stretches for a minimum of 10 seconds and up to 60 seconds; repeat each two to four times.
- Give tighter areas extra attention, with more duration and frequency.
- Breathe slowly and deeply through the stretches, maintaining an even ratio of inhalations to exhalations.

Flexibility is an integral part of your overall fitness equation. Given the movements involved in swimming, biking, and running, stretching is especially important for those training for a triathlon. Flexible knees and hips extend better during your cycling stroke. Pliable shoulders help you in swimming. Supple hamstrings aid on the bike. Flexible quadriceps facilitate running efficiency. Static or slow, steady stretching at low intensity is the most favorable technique you can employ. Engaging in a regular stretching program reaps many benefits such as increased performance, decreased recovery time, and reduced risk of injury.

Standing Quadriceps Stretch

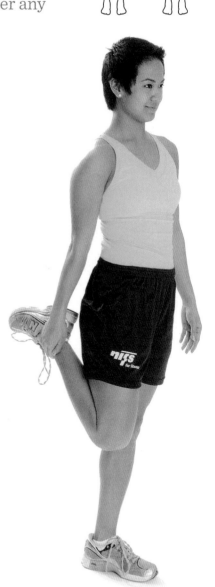

This stretch will target your quadriceps (large muscle group at the front of your upper leg), which is important after any long or fast bike or run.

1. Stand up, holding onto something for balance with one hand if necessary. With your free hand, grasp your corresponding upper foot and ankle, and bring your heel toward your buttocks. Keep your knees adjacent to one another.

2. Maintain alignment as you pull back, stretching your quad muscle.

3. Hold for 30 to 60 seconds and then switch legs.

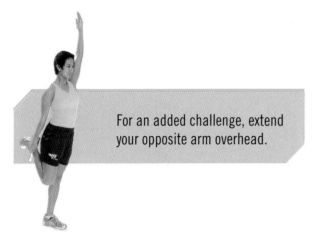

For an added challenge, extend your opposite arm overhead.

Hamstring Rope Stretch

Reaching down to touch your toes is the most basic way to stretch your hamstrings (the back of your upper leg). This will get the same stretch done with less stress on your back.

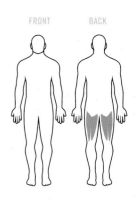

FRONT   BACK

1. Lie on your back with one leg extended. Loop a rope or towel around your other foot and hold one end of the rope in each hand.

2. Keep your extended leg flat on the floor as you bring your other leg up and back.

3. Press the heel of your raised leg up toward the ceiling and feel the stretch in the back of your leg. Pull your leg to your torso as far as your hamstrings allow.

4. Hold for 30 to 60 seconds and then switch legs.

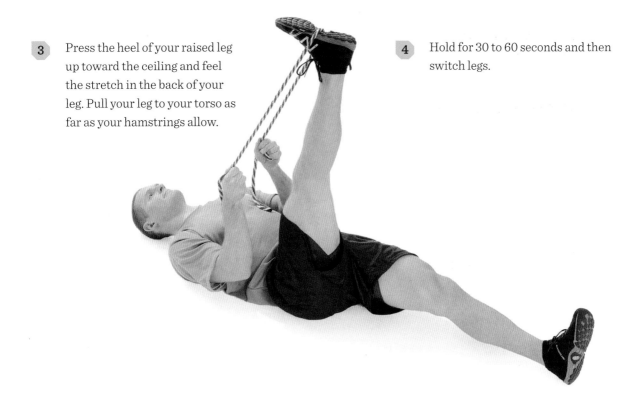

Standing Calf Stretch

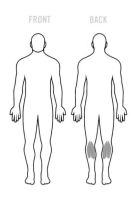

FRONT   BACK

This will stretch your calf (the back of the lower part of your leg).

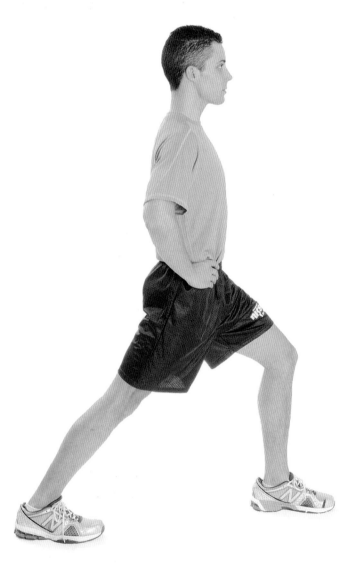

1   Stand with your feet shoulder width apart, one foot planted about a foot in front of the other.

2   Keep both feet flat on the ground as you shift your weight forward and bend your front leg. Feel the stretch in the back of your straight leg.

3   Hold for 30 to 60 seconds and then switch legs.

Standing Piriformis Stretch

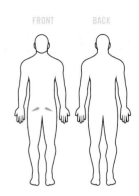

The piriformis is a small, pear-shaped muscle located deep in the hip behind the glutes and close to the sciatic nerve. It is a rotator muscle that helps rotate your leg out. Stretching the piriformis should never be skipped. It is a common site of injury and pain for triathletes.

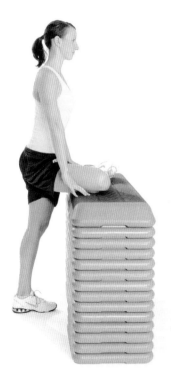
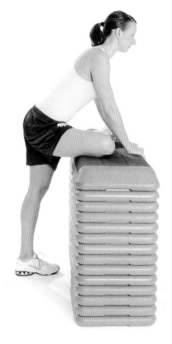
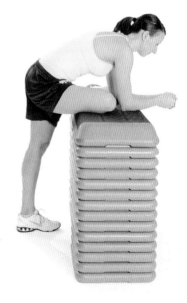

1   Lay your right leg as flat as possible on a platform just below hip height. Bend your leg inward so your foot is pointed to the left. Your right knee should be in line with the foot.

2   Engage your core, keep your back flat, and slowly bend forward at the hips. Move as far forward as is comfortable until you feel the stretch in your hips and glutes.

3   Press your knee down toward the surface, then relax and move further into the stretch.

4   Hold for 30 to 60 seconds and then switch sides.

Standing Hip Flexor Stretch

The hip flexors are a group of muscles that allow you to lift your knees and bend at the waist. Increasing their range of motion with stretching improves overall athletic performance.

1 Stand with your feet staggered in a lunge position with your right leg forward and knees slightly bent. Keep your shoulders square, maintain good posture, and place your hands on your hips.

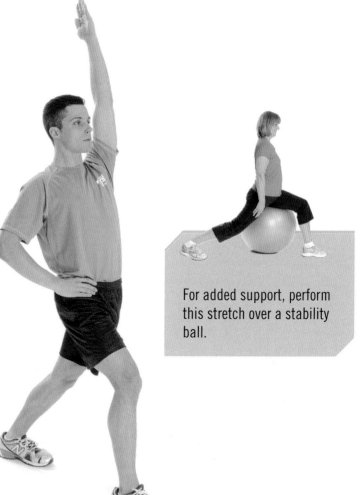

2 Move into the stretch by gently lowering your front knee while raising your opposite side arm overhead. Drop your hips and put most of your weight on the front leg. Open the back hip until you feel tension in the left thigh and right hip. Drop your hips and feel the stretch.

3 Hold for 30 to 60 seconds and then switch legs.

For added support, perform this stretch over a stability ball.

Seated Leg Crossover

This stretch targets the lower back and the hip flexors.

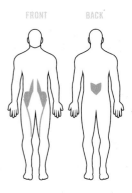

FRONT   BACK

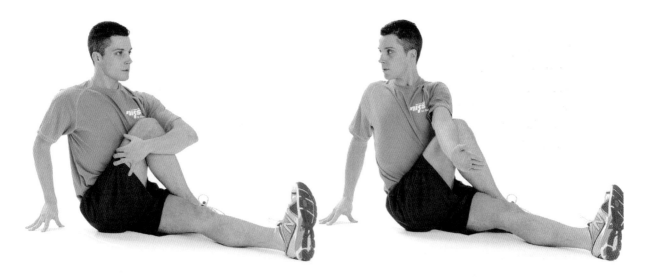

1. Sit tall on the floor with your left leg extended. Bend your right leg and place your right foot on the outside of your left knee. Place your right hand on the floor behind your right buttock for support.

2. While twisting to your right, bring your left arm across your right knee, and gaze out over your right shoulder. Apply passive or gentle pressure between your left upper arm and right knee.

3. Hold for 30 to 60 seconds and then switch sides.

Cat and Camel

This stretch will be a welcome addition to your routine, especially after a long bike ride. Your back and core will thank you.

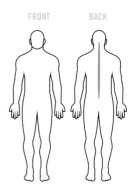

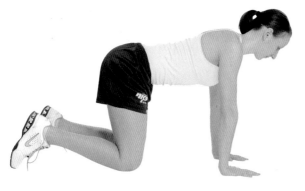

1. Begin on your hands and knees with your back flat, your hands directly below your shoulders, and your knees below your hips. Keep a slight bend in your elbows with your fingers facing forward.

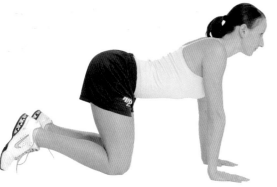

2. Slowly arch your spine downward by releasing your hips. Exhale as you press down as far as is comfortable.

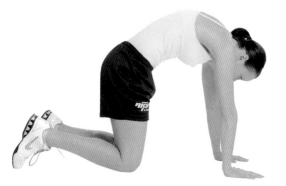

3. Gently round your back. Feel the stretch throughout your spine as you lengthen your shoulders and back.

4. Hold for 30 to 60 seconds.

Lying Chest Lift (Cobra)

This stretch will continue to work on your back muscles, but will utilize more of your body weight to push the stretch further than Cat and Camel.

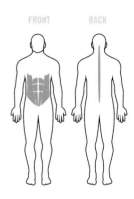

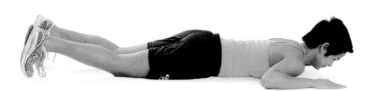

1 Lie on your stomach and place your hands shoulder width apart on the floor near your eyes. Keep your toes on the floor.

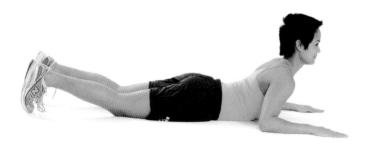

2 Raise your upper body while keeping your hips and lower body in contact with the floor. Feel the stretch open up your core.

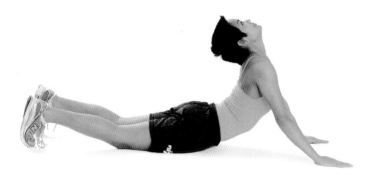

3 Extend your arms as fully as you can. Finish with your neck long and your head high.

4 Hold for 30 to 60 seconds.

Overhead Triceps Rope Stretch

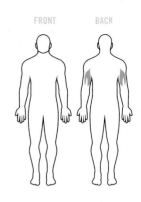

FRONT   BACK

This stretch targets the triceps, the muscles on the back of your upper arm. You'll need a rope or even a sturdy shirt or towel.

1 Stand with your feet shoulder width apart. Holding a rope, reach your left hand over your left shoulder. Grab the rope with your opposite hand near your lower back.

2 Apply tension by pulling down the rope. Find a point where you feel the stretch in the back of the upper arm.

3 Hold for 30 to 60 seconds and then switch arms.

Alternatively, you can raise a bent arm, elbow up, with the palm of that hand resting on your back. Use your opposite hand to pull the elbow in tighter.

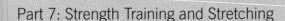

Standing Wall Chest Stretch

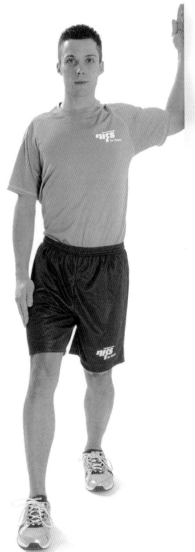

This exercise will open up your chest muscles and stretch your pectorals. If you've just spent a long time in the aero position on your bike, you will love this.

1. Stand sideways next to a wall with your left arm resting against the wall at a 90-degree angle.

2. Maintain the arm position and slowly take a step forward with the right leg. Gently twist your upper body away from the wall.

3. Hold for 30 to 60 seconds and then switch sides.

Bent Arm Crossover

This stretch will target your triceps and your shoulders.

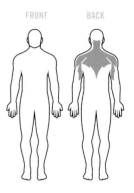

FRONT   BACK

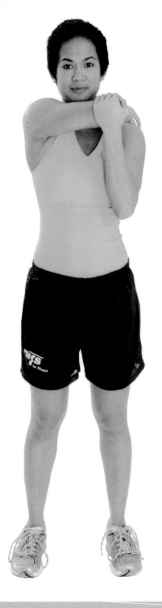

1   Stand with your feet shoulder width apart. Relax your shoulders and let them drop down. Bring your right arm across your chest, parallel to the floor, and over your left shoulder.

2   Using your left hand, apply gentle pressure to your right arm, pressing it toward your body.

3   Hold for 30 to 60 seconds and then switch arms.

Side Neck Stretch

In all three legs of the triathlon, you'll use your neck muscles: to breathe while swimming; to keep your head up while biking; to stabilize while running. Make sure to stretch your neck slowly.

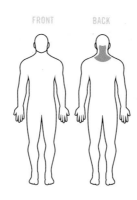

FRONT BACK

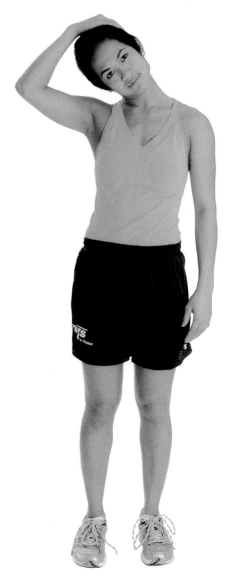

1. Stand or sit erect with your eyes facing forward. Place your right hand on top of your head and slowly bring your right ear to your shoulder, applying very gentle pressure with your hand. You should feel the muscles on the left side of your neck stretch and lengthen.

2. Hold for 30 to 60 seconds, then return to the starting position and repeat the stretch on the opposite side.

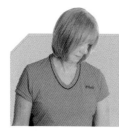

You can also perform this stretch just by moving your neck, without the assistance from your hand and arm.

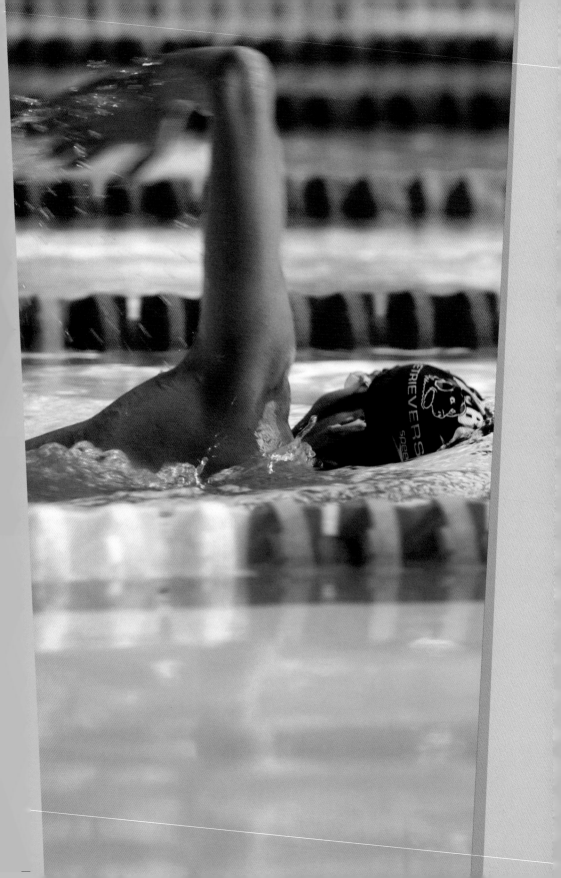

Triathlon Training Programs

The training programs in the upcoming pages will get you ready and where you need to be for your triathlon. As you'll see, we outline exactly what to do each day. There will be weeks of building longer workouts, followed by rest days and weeks. Trust the program.

In order to determine the actual dates associated with each workout on the schedule, match up your race date with the "race day" on the schedule, and work backward.

Once you've started the program, if you miss a day, or end up having to rearrange some (or even many!) of the workouts, do not panic. A successful triathlete needs to be able to adapt, adjust, and overcome. You will be prepared. Go for it!

Training Program Philosophy

There is no exact science to a training program. What might work for your friend may not work as well for you. The programs in this book are meant to be guidelines. Allow yourself flexibility if your schedule gets too hectic. Listen to your body and adjust your program based on how you feel. Use common sense at all times and you'll be fine.

Program Organization

Six days a week, you will have a bike, swim, or run workout—or a workout that includes all three. The workouts may be broken out into Warm-up, Workout, and Cooldown, or they may simply indicate how many minutes to spend in the water or on the road. Sometimes workouts are given in terms of intervals. For example:

Run:	8×2-minute intervals	Z3	1 minute rest

This means you run for two minutes, during which you should be working hard enough so your heart rate is in Zone 3. At the end of the 2-minute interval, you back off the pace and recover for 1 minute. You then repeat the entire process seven more times for a total of eight intervals.

The longest workouts occur on Days 6 and 7. These workouts should be completed on the weekends, or on the days when you have the most free time in your schedule. Adjust your training program accordingly.

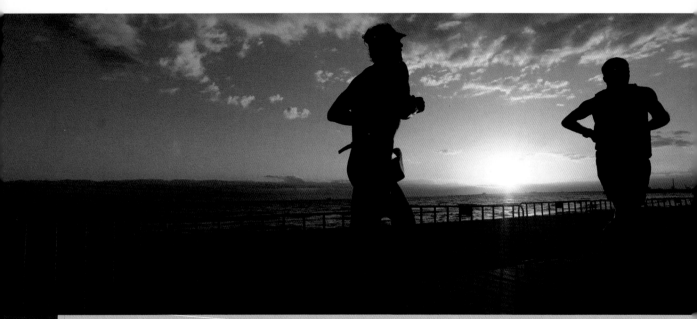

Part 8: Triathlon Training Programs

Swim Notes

Swim workouts may be given in time or distance. Because pools can be measured in yards or meters, the distance workouts do not include a unit of measure. For example:

Swim: 8×100   Z2   30 seconds rest

This means that you swim 100 meters (or yards) with your heart rate in Zone 2. At the end of 100 meters, you rest for 30 seconds, and then repeat seven more times. Try to find a pool that is at least 20 meters (or yards) long so you have enough room to stretch out your form.

Bike Notes

Some bike workouts include drills that are intended to be performed using an indoor trainer. You can try to do some of the suggested workouts on the road, but if you do, be sure you do it in an area with very little traffic. Do not attempt the single leg drills (SLDs) out on the road as it could cause you to lose balance. If you don't have a trainer, we suggest skipping the BGD/SGD/SLD workouts and completing hill intervals on that day.

Also, unless otherwise noted, your cadence on the bike should be somewhere between 80 and 100 RPMs.

Strength Training and Stretching Notes

Strength training is not explicitly included on the training schedule, but we recommend adding some weight lifting to your workouts two to three days each week. Try to stretch for a few minutes after each workout to improve flexibility and prevent injury.

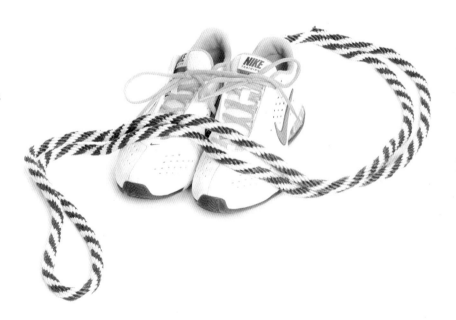

Training Intensity

Each workout is labeled as Z1, Z2, Z3, or Z4. These codes stand for Zone 1, Zone 2, Zone 3, and Zone 4. The zones indicate the level of intensity at which you should be working out, using your heart rate and rate of perceived exertion.

Description	Zone	Percent of Max Heart Rate	Rate of Perceived Exertion (RPE)	Abbreviation
Active recovery	1	55 to 65	12 to 13	Z1
Endurance	2	65 to 75	13 to 15	Z2
Resistance	3	75 to 85	15 to 16	Z3
Threshold	4	85 to 90	16 to 18	Z4

Zone 1 is used early in the training program as well as for active recovery workouts.

Zone 2 is great for building aerobic capacity.

Zone 3 takes it to the next level and incorporates aerobic work while it flirts with anaerobic training.

Zone 4 is an intense effort at anaerobic threshold. Your fitness level should be at a sufficient capacity before entering this zone. Ample recovery should always be taken following such a workout to allow for effective fitness absorption. Zone 4 is not to be used at the beginning of a training program.

Calculating Your Target Heart Rate

To accurately evaluate the intensity of your workout, you'll need to know your target heart rate and RPE (rate of perceived exertion). To calculate your target heart rate for each zone, use the following formula:

Target heart rate (THR) = (220 – age) × desired intensity percent

For example, here's how to find the Zone 3 intensity for a 20-year-old. Remember, Zone 3 is 75 to 85 percent of your target heart rate.

Lower THR = (220 – 20) × 0.75 = 150

Upper THR = (220 – 20) × 0.85 = 170

For this individual, Zone 3 range is 150-170 beats per minute.

Once you've calculated your target heart rate, use a heart rate monitor to check your beats per minute.

Determining Your RPE

A second method of intensity training is the Rate of Perceived Exertion (RPE). This is a more subjective approach developed by Dr. Gunnar Borg. It is also referred to as the Borg Scale. The Borg Scale takes into consideration what you are experiencing and perceiving: psychological, musculoskeletal, and environmental factors, as well as overall fatigue. The original scale ranges from 6-20. Each degree of the scale corresponds to heart rate. A 6 on the scale represents 60 beats per minute, a 130 represents 130 beats per minute, and so on.

Each number carries an associated intensity characterization. For example, 13 (in the middle of the scale) translates to "somewhat hard." Over time, you will learn how each number correlates to effort. It will become natural for you to feel what a 13 is, and if your schedule calls for it, maintain the right level of intensity.

Rate of Perceived Exertion

6	
7	Very, very light
8	
9	Very light
10	
11	Fairly light
12	
13	Somewhat hard
14	
15	Hard
16	
17	Very hard
18	
19	Very, very hard
20	

The Right Mixture

Ideally, you will learn to strike a balance between heart rate intensities and RPE. This is important because sometimes there's a deviation between the "standard" heart rate and age that can impact the training zones. For example, research has demonstrated that older adults may have significantly higher max heart rates. Women have also been found to generally have higher heart rates at the same levels of work output.

It's best to use the heart rate formula in combination with the RPE scale. If you find you deviate from the formula, make the adjustments to your training zone numbers. For example, you may find your heart rate is in Zone 2, but you only feel you're working in RPE matching moderate output, 12-13.

Extreme heat stress and elevation can skew heart rate, too. Both scenarios can result in above-normal heart rates for a given output. RPE is the better indicator in such examples.

Program Overview

Sprint-Distance Training

Although it varies, a sprint-distance triathlon typically consists of a half-mile (.8 km) swim, a 12- to 14-mile (19-22.5 km) bike and a 3.1-mile (5 km) run. Depending on your fitness level, you'll need 6 to 14 weeks to train for a race of this length. Even if you're comfortable with all three of these sports and feel like you could just "wing it" on race day (which is not recommended), following a program will make you more prepared on race day and help things go more smoothly.

Our schedule is 12 weeks long and includes six days of training each week. Don't be afraid to shift the workouts a bit as necessary to fit your schedule and lifestyle. Training for a sprint triathlon should not stress you out or feel like a full time job. That said, put in the time so you will feel confident and be ready.

Olympic-Distance Training

An Olympic-distance triathlon consists of a 0.93-mile (1.5 km) swim, a 24.8-mile (40 km) bike, and a 6.2-mile (10 km) run. You'll want to allow at least 8 to 16 weeks to prepare for an Olympic-distance triathlon.

Our Olympic-distance training schedule is 16 weeks long and includes six days of training each week. You can rearrange the workouts as needed to fit your schedule, but do your best to stay on track and don't skip too many. You'll need to train properly to have a successful race.

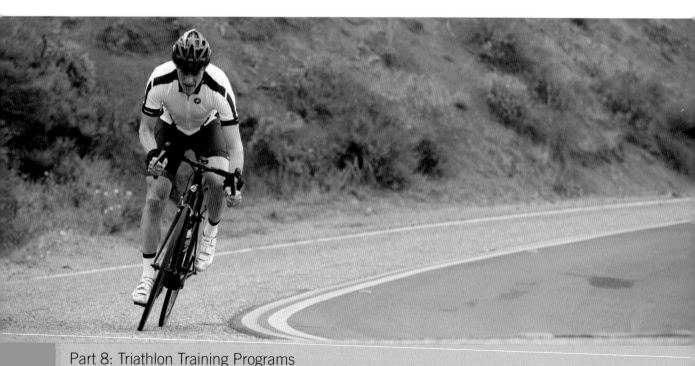

Baseline Fitness

Before you start, you should be able to swim from one end of the pool to the other without stopping. If you're not there yet, then enroll in a beginner's class and work on your stroke a bit. You should also be able to ride a bicycle, although the distance isn't too important. Many beginners choose to do a combination of running and walking to train for the "run" portion of the race. This is fine! You should be able to walk/run at least two miles before you begin training for a sprint-distance triathlon, and at least three to four miles before you begin training for an Olympic-distance triathlon.

Target Times

As you train, you are going to build up to the following durations:

Sprint-Distance

Swim: 25 minutes

Bike: 75 minutes

Run: 60 minutes

Olympic-Distance

Swim: 60 minutes

Bike: 150 minutes

Run: 90 minutes

The length of time you spend working out each day will slowly build as you get further into your program. Some weeks are "recovery weeks," and the duration of workouts will be reduced. Allow yourself the break. Training duration is also reduced as you get near race day (this is called *tapering*). You may feel like you want to go longer, but allow yourself the rest. Your body will thank you!

Drills

These training programs include specific technique drills for each of the three disciplines. Try to follow the workouts specifically laid out for swimming when possible, and do the drills when suggested for running. For biking, don't worry if you aren't able to incorporate as many drills as we suggest. Most people will be able to find a hill to do some repeats, but do not worry about buying an expensive indoor trainer to do the other drills. They are more of a "nice to have" than a necessity. Even if you skip all of the biking drills, you'll still be prepared for the race.

Diet and Nutrition

During your training, you'll find that your appetite will increase (sometimes substantially). This is normal. You don't need to make radical changes to your diet as you train, but be sure to give your body the fuel it needs. Have healthy snacks available for pre- and post-workout nutrition. Products designed for athletes are fine, but you can get all the calories and nutrients you need from whole foods such as fruits, vegetables, lean proteins, nuts, and grains.

Sprint Training: Week 1

	COMPONENT			ZONE	REST	NOTES
DAY 1	**Swim:**	Warm-up	4×50	Z1	15 seconds	Strong swimmer: Increase each workout rep length by 25.
		Workout	6×75	Z2	15 seconds	
		Cooldown	6×25	Z1	10 seconds	
		TOTAL	800			
DAY 2	**Run:**		30 minutes	Z1 or Z2		
DAY 3	**Bike:**		45 minutes	Z1		
DAY 4	**Swim:**	Warm-up	5×50	Z1	15 seconds	Strong swimmer: Increase warm-up by 1 rep, increase workout by 2 reps, and decrease rest times by 5 seconds.
		Workout	6×100	Z2	15 seconds	
		Cooldown	6×25	Z1	15 seconds	
		TOTAL	1,000			
DAY 5	**Rest**					
DAY 6	**Bike:**		45 minutes	Z1 or Z2		Try to start your run within 5 to 10 minutes after the ride, but slow down and take it easy if you find it difficult to keep your heart rate or breathing under control.
	Run:		10 minutes	Z1		
	Swim:	(optional)	10 to 15 minutes, drills or laps			
DAY 7	**Run:**		37 minutes	Z1		

Sprint Training: Week 2

	COMPONENT			ZONE	REST	NOTES
DAY 1	**Swim:**	Warm-Up	4×50	Z1	15 seconds	Strong swimmer: Do 16×50 for your workout.
		Workout	10×50	Z2	15 seconds	
			10×25	Z2	10 seconds	
		Cooldown	2×100	Z1	10 seconds	
		TOTAL	1,000			
DAY 2	**Run:**	Warm-up	15 minutes	Z1		
		Workout	10 minutes of pick-ups, alternate 1 minute fast, 1 minute recovery	Z2		
		Cooldown	5 to 10 minutes	Z1		
DAY 3	**Bike:**		45 minutes	Z1		
DAY 4	**Swim:**	Warm-Up	6×50	Z1	15 seconds	Strong swimmer: Do 6×150 for your workout and decrease rest times by 5 seconds.
		Workout	2×150	Z2	15 seconds	
			3×100	Z2	10 seconds	
		Cooldown	4×50	Z1	10 seconds	
		Total	1,100			
DAY 5	**Rest**					
DAY 6	**Bike:**		55 minutes	Z1 or Z2		Do your 10-minute run immediately after you finish your bike ride Remember to set up all the gear you'll need for your run before you head out on your bike.
	Run:		10-minute T-run	Z1		
	Swim:	(optional)	15 minutes of drills or laps			
DAY 7	**Run:**		40 minutes	Z1		The long run increases by 3 minutes from last week. Keep the pace relaxed, and utilize the "talk test" to make sure you're not pushing too hard.

Sprint Training: Week 3

	COMPONENT			ZONE	REST	NOTES
DAY 1	**Swim:**	Warm-up	2×100	Z1	15 seconds	For warm-up: Do 100 swim, 100 drills. Strong swimmer: Increase workout set by 2 reps and decrease rest by 5 seconds.
		Workout	7×100	Z2	20 seconds	
		Cooldown	4×50	Z1	10 seconds	
		TOTAL	1,100			
DAY 2	**Run:**	Warm-up	10 minutes, 4 accelerations	Z1		Strong runner: Speed workout with some accelerations and drills.
		Workout	15 minutes of			
			3×2 - minute intervals	Z2	3 minutes	
		Drills	1×25 per leg of each drill			
		Cooldown	10 minutes	Z1		
DAY 3	**Bike:**	Warm-up	15 minutes	Z1	2 minutes	If you don't feel like you have enough recovery time between intervals, you may be pushing too hard. Pull back.
		Workout	20 minutes of			
			4×3 - minute intervals	Z2	2 minutes	
		Cooldown	10 minutes	Z1		
DAY 4	**Swim:**	Warm-up	3×100	Z1	15 seconds	Strong swimmer: Do 8×100 and 4×50.
		Workout	8×50	Z2	10 seconds	
			4×100	Z2	15 seconds	
		Cooldown	4×50	Z1	10 seconds	
		TOTAL	1,300			
DAY 5	**Rest**					
DAY 6	**Bike:**		65 minutes	Z1 or Z2		Bring nutrition for the bike ride. Begin your T-run immediately after biking.
	Run:		10 minute T-run	Z1		
	Swim:	(optional)	10 to 15 minutes, drills or laps			
DAY 7	**Run:**		45 minutes	Z1		It's okay to take a break and walk if you need to.

Sprint Training: Week 4

	COMPONENT			ZONE	REST	NOTES
DAY 1	**Swim:**	Warm-up	4×50	Z1	15 seconds	Strong swimmer: Increase each workout rep length by 25.
		Workout	6×75	Z2	15 seconds	
		Cooldown	6×25	Z1	10 seconds	
		TOTAL	800			
DAY 2	**Run:**	Warm-up	10 minutes, 4 accelerations	Z1		Strong runner: Push yourself during the fartlek run. Stay anywhere below Z4 when you're picking up the pace.
		Workout	15 minutes of fartlek	Z2 to Z3		
		Drills	1×25 per leg of each drill			
		Cooldown	10 minutes	Z1		
DAY 3	**Bike:**	Warm-up	10 minutes	Z1		
		Workout	15 minutes of 3×3-minute intervals	Z2	2 minutes	
		Cooldown	10 minutes	Z1		
DAY 4	**Swim:**	Warm-Up	6×50	Z1	15 seconds	Strong swimmer: Do 20×50 as main workout.
		Workout	5×50	Z2	15 seconds	
			10×25	Z3	10 seconds	
		Cooldown	2×100	Z1	15 seconds	
		TOTAL	1000			
DAY 5	**Rest**					
DAY 6	**Bike:**		50 minutes	Z1 or Z2		Begin your T-run immediately after biking.
	Run:		10-minute T-run	Z1 or Z2		
DAY 7	**Run:**		35 minutes	Z2		

Sprint Training: Week 5

	COMPONENT			ZONE	REST	NOTES
DAY 1	**Swim:**	Warm-up	5×50	Z1	15 seconds	After your swim, hop on your bike to get the feel for that transition.
		Workout	3×100	Z2	15 seconds	
			3×200	Z2	25 seconds	
		Cooldown	2×100	Z1	10 seconds	
		TOTAL	1,350			
	Bike:		10 minutes	Z1		
DAY 2	**Run:**	Warm-up	15 minutes, 6 accelerations	Z1		Strong runner: Reduce warm-up and increase tempo run by 5 min each.
		Workout	10-minute tempo run	Z2 or Z3		
		Drills	1×25 per leg of each drill			
		Cooldown	10 minutes	Z1		
DAY 3	**Bike:**	Warm-up	15 minutes	Z1		Alternative: Find a steep hill and do 4 minutes uphill, 2 minutes downhill, and repeat 3 times.
		Workout	4×30-second SLDs	Z2 or Z3		
			2 minutes	Z1		
			5×2 - minute LGDs	Z2	1 minute	
		Cooldown	10 minutes	Z1		
DAY 4	**Swim:**	Warm-up	3×100	Z1	15 seconds	Strong swimmer: Add 5 more 50s to the set and decrease the rest for the 100s to 10 seconds.
		Workout	10×50	Z3	10 seconds	
			5×100	Z3	15 seconds	
		Cooldown	4×50	Z1	10 seconds	
		TOTAL	1,500			
DAY 5	**Rest**					
DAY 6	**Bike:**		70 minutes	Z1 or Z2		Do your T-run run right after you finish your bike ride.
	Run:		15-minute T-run	Z1		
	Swim:	(optional)	10 to 15 minutes, drills or laps			
DAY 7	**Run:**		45 minutes	Z1		

Sprint Training: Week 6

	COMPONENT			ZONE	REST	NOTES
DAY 1	**Swim:**	Warm-up	6×50	Z1	15 seconds	Strong swimmer: Add a 200 and decrease the rest for the 100s to 10 seconds.
		Workout	6×100	Z2	15 seconds	
			2×200	Z2	20 seconds	
		Cooldown	5×50	Z1	15 seconds	
		TOTAL	1,550			
DAY 2	**Run:**	Warm-up	10 minutes, 6 accelerations	Z1		
		Workout	15-minute interval set;			
			2 min pickup, 1 min easy	Z3		
		Drills	1×25 per leg of each drill			
		Cooldown	10 minutes	Z1		
	Swim:	(optional)	20 minutes in open water			
DAY 3	**Bike:**	Warm-up	15 minutes	Z1		Alternative bike: Do 4 minutes uphill (hard), then 2 minutes downhill; repeat 4 times.
		Workout	6×30-second SLDs			
			2 minutes	Z1		
			5×2-minute LGDs	Z2	1 minute	
		Cooldown	10 minutes	Z1		
	Run:	(optional)	10-minute T-run			
	Swim:	(optional)	12 to 20 minutes in open water			
DAY 4	**Swim:**	Warm-up	3×100	Z1	15 seconds	Strong swimmer: Add an extra 100 and an extra 200 to your workout.
		Workout	8×50	Z3	10 seconds	
			5×100	Z2 to Z3	15 seconds	
			2×200	Z2	20 seconds	
		Cooldown	2×100	Z1	10 seconds	
		TOTAL	1,800			
DAY 5	**Rest**					
DAY 6	**Bike:**		82 minutes	Z1 or Z2		Begin your T-run immediately after biking.
	Run:		15-minute T-run			
	Swim:	(optional)	drills, laps, or open-water swim			
	Run:		50 minutes	Z1		

Sprint Training: Week 7

	COMPONENT			ZONE	REST	NOTES
DAY 1	**Swim:**	Warm-up	3×100	Z1	20 seconds	Strong swimmer: Add a 200 to your workout and decrease the rest by 5 seconds.
		Workout	6×200	Z2	25 seconds	
		Cooldown	6×50	Z1	10 seconds	
		TOTAL	1,800			
DAY 2	**Run:**	Warm-up	10 minutes, 4 accelerations	Z1		
		Workout	15-minute interval set;			
			3 minutes pickup,			
			2 minutes easy	Z2 to Z3		
		Drills	2×20 per leg of each drill			
		Cooldown	10 minutes	Z1		
DAY 3	**Bike:**	Warm-up	15 minutes	Z1		Alternative bike: 4 minutes uphill (hard), then 2 minutes downhill; repeat 5 times.
		Workout	4×1-minute SGDs	Z3	1 minute	
			5×2-minute LGDs	Z3	1 minute	
			4×1-minute SGDs	Z3	1 minute	
		Cooldown	10 minutes	Z1		
	Run:	(optional)	10-minute T-run			
DAY 4	**Swim:**	Warm-Up	3×100	Z1	15 seconds	Strong swimmer: Add an extra 100 and an extra 200 to the workout.
		Workout	8×50	Z3	10 seconds	
			5×100	Z2 to Z3	15 seconds	
			3×200	Z2	20 seconds	
		Cooldown	2×100	Z1	10 seconds	
		TOTAL	1,800			
DAY 5	**Rest**					
DAY 6	**Bike:**		90 minutes	Z1 or Z2		
	Run:		15-minute T-run	Z1		
	Swim:	(optional)	15 minutes, drills or laps			
DAY 7	**Run:**		55 minutes	Z1		

Sprint Training: Week 8

	COMPONENT			ZONE	REST	NOTES
DAY 1	**Swim:**	Warm-up	6×50	Z1	15 seconds	Strong swimmer: Increase 200s and decrease 100s, 1 for 1 (e.g., 3×100, 4×200) up to 7×200.
		Workout	4×100	Z2	15 seconds	
			3×200	Z2	25 seconds	
		Cooldown	4×50	Z1	10 seconds	
		TOTAL	1,500			
DAY 2	**Run:**	Warm-up	10 minutes, 6 accelerations	Z1		Keep your tempo run steady throughout.
		Workout	10-minute tempo run	Z2 to Z3		
		Drills	2×25 per leg of each drill			
		Cooldown	10 minutes	Z1		
DAY 3	**Bike:**	Warm-up	15 minutes	Z1		Strong cyclist: Increase interval length to 4 minutes and reduce recovery to 1 minute.
		Workout	5×3-minute intervals	Z3	2 minutes	
		Cooldown	10 minutes	Z1		
	Run:	(optional)	10-minute T-run			
DAY 4	**Swim:**	Warm-up	2×100	Z1	15 seconds	Strong swimmer: Do 7×200 instead of 10×100; keep rest at 15 seconds.
		Workout	10×100	Z2	15 seconds	
		Cooldown	4×50	Z1	10 seconds	
		TOTAL	1,400			
DAY 5	**Rest**					
DAY 6	**Bike:**		60 minutes	Z1 or Z2		Begin your T-run immediately after the bike ride.
	Run:		10-minute T-run	Z1		
	Swim:	(optional)	15 minutes, drills or laps			
DAY 7	**Run:**		40 minutes	Z1		

Sprint Training: Week 9

	COMPONENT			ZONE	REST	NOTES
DAY 1	**Swim:**	Warm-up	3×100	Z1	15 seconds	Strong swimmer: Add a 300 and decrease the rest time by 5 seconds.
		Workout	4×300	Z2	30 seconds	
		Cooldown	6×50	Z1	10 seconds	
		TOTAL	1,800			
DAY 2	**Run:**	Warm-up	10 minutes, 6 accelerations	Z1		Strong runner: Increase pickup to 3 minutes, and give yourself 45 seconds to recover.
		Workout	6×2-minute intervals	Z2 to Z3	30 seconds	
		Drills	2×30 per leg of each drill			
		Cooldown	10 minutes	Z1		
DAY 3	**Bike:**	Warm-up	15 minutes	Z1		Alternative bike: After the warm-up, do a 10-minute interval in Z3 to Z4; recover for 5 minutes, and repeat.
		Workout	5×1 minute SGDs	Z3	1 minute	
			2×2 minute LGDs	Z3	1 minute	
			5×1 minute SGDs	Z4		
		Cooldown	10 minutes	Z1		
	Run:	(optional)	10-minute T-run	Z1		
DAY 4	**Swim:**	Warm-up	3×100	Z1	15 seconds	Strong swimmer: Make each consecutive rep within a given set faster.
		Workout	7×100	Z3	15 seconds	
			1×100	Z1		
			7×50	Z3	10 seconds	
			1×100	Z1		
			7×25	Z4	5 seconds	
		Cooldown	1×300	Z1		
		TOTAL	2,025			
DAY 5	**Rest**					
DAY 6	**Bike:**		75 minutes	Z1 or Z2		Don't forget your fluids and energy.
	Run:		10-minute T-run			
	Swim:	(optional)	15 minutes, drills or laps			
DAY 7	**Run:**		60 minutes	Z2		

Sprint Training: Week 10

	COMPONENT			ZONE	REST	NOTES
DAY 1	**Swim:**	Warm-up	8×25	Z1	5 seconds	Strong swimmer: Add a fast 50 (Z3) between the 500s (500-50-500-50-500) and decrease the rest time by 20 seconds.
		Workout	3×500	Z2	60 seconds	
		Cooldown	6×50	Z1	10 seconds	
		TOTAL	2,000			
DAY 2	**Run:**	Warm-up	10 minutes, 8 accelerations	Z1		
		Workout	15-minute fartlek	Z3 to Z4		
		Drills	2×30 per leg of each drill			
		Cooldown	10 minutes	Z1		
DAY 3	**Bike:**	Warm-up	15 minutes	Z1		Alternative bike: Do hill intervals of 4 minutes uphill, 2 minutes downhill. Repeat 5 times.
		Workout	5×4 minutes of drills	Z3 or Z4	1 minute	
		Cooldown	10 minutes	Z1		
	Run:	(optional)	10-minute T-run			
DAY 4	**Swim:**	Warm-up	3×100	Z1	15 seconds	Strong swimmer: Add an extra set of 75s at the end of the workout.
		Workout	3×75	Z3 to Z4	15 seconds	
			1×250	Z2 to Z3	15 seconds	
			Repeat 3 times			
		Cooldown	300	Z1		
		TOTAL	2,025			
DAY 5	**Rest**					
DAY 6	**Bike:**	65 minutes	Z1 or Z2			
	Run:	10-minute T-run	Z1			
	Swim:	(optional)	15 minutes, drills or laps			
DAY 7	**Run:**		50 minutes	Z2		

Sprint Training: Week 11

	COMPONENT			ZONE	REST	NOTES
DAY 1	**Swim:**	Warm-up	2×100	Z1	15 seconds	Strong swimmer: Add a 200 and decrease the rest time for the 100s to 10 seconds.
		Workout	6×100	Z3	15 seconds	
			3×200	Z2	25 seconds	
		Cooldown	4×50	Z1	15 seconds	
		TOTAL	1,600			
DAY 2	**Run:**	Warm-up	10 minutes, 5 accelerations	Z1		Strong runner: Extend your tempo run to 12-15 minutes.
		Workout	10-minute tempo run			
		Drills	2×15 per leg of each drill			
		Cooldown	10 minutes	Z1		
DAY 3	**Bike:**	Warm-up	15 minutes	Z1		
		Workout	4×3-minute intervals	Z3 or Z4	2 minutes	
		Cooldown	10 minutes	Z1		
	Run:	(optional)	10-minute T-run			
DAY 4	**Swim:**	Warm-up	4×100	Z1	15 seconds	Strong swimmer: Add 4×50 to the workout.
		Workout	16×50	Z2 to Z4	10 seconds	
		Cooldown	6×50	Z1	10 seconds	
		TOTAL	1,500			
DAY 5	**Rest**					
DAY 6	**Bike:**		55 minutes	Z1 or Z2		
	Run:		10 minute T-run	Z1		
	Swim:	(optional)	10 to 15 minutes, drills or laps	Z1		
DAY 7	**Run:**		40 minutes	Z1		

Sprint Training: Week 12

	COMPONENT			ZONE	REST	NOTES
DAY 1	**Swim:**	Warm-up	2×100	Z1	15 seconds	Strong swimmer: Add a 200 and decrease the rest time for the 100s to 15 seconds.
		Workout	3×100	Z3	20 seconds	
			4×200	Z2	25 seconds	
		Cooldown	4×50	Z1	10 seconds	
		TOTAL	1,500			
DAY 2	**Run:**	Warm-Up	10 minutes, 4 accelerations	Z1		
		Workout	5×30 seconds fast, 1 minute easy between	Z3 to Z4		
		Drills	1×20 per leg of each drill			
		Cooldown	7 minutes, 30 seconds	Z1		
DAY 3	**Bike:**	Warm-up	15 minutes	Z1		
		Workout	4×2-minute intervals of high resistance/fast spinning	Z3 or Z4	3 minutes	
		Cooldown	10 minutes	Z1		
	Run:	(optional)	10-minute T-run			
DAY 4	**Swim:**	Warm-up	2×100	Z1	15 seconds	
		Workout	1×200	Z2	15 seconds	
			2×100	Z2	15 seconds	
			3×75	Z3	15 seconds	
			4×50	Z3	15 seconds	
			5×25	Z4	15 seconds	
		Cooldown	5×50	Z1	10 seconds	
		TOTAL	1,500			
DAY 5	**Rest**					
DAY 6	**Swim:**		10 minutes	Z1		If possible, do your workouts where you'll be racing tomorrow.
	Bike:		30 minutes	Z2		
	Run:		15 minutes	Z1		
DAY 7	**RACE DAY!**					

Olympic-Distance Training: Week 1

	COMPONENT			ZONE	REST	NOTES
DAY 1	**Swim:**	Warm-up	4×50	Z1	15 seconds	
		Workout	6×100	Z2	15 seconds	
		Cooldown	4×50	Z1	15 seconds	
		TOTAL	1,000			
DAY 2	**Run:**		25 minutes	Z1 or Z2		
DAY 3	**Bike:**		35 minutes	Z1 or Z2		
DAY 4	**Swim:**	Warm-up	5×50	Z1	15 seconds	Incorporate at least three drills in your warm-up.
		Workout	6×100	Z2	15 seconds	
		Cooldown	4×75	Z1	10 seconds	
		TOTAL	1,150			
DAY 5	**Rest**					
DAY 6	**Bike:**		65 minutes	Z1 or Z2		Set up all the running gear you need before you head out on your bike. After you finish your bike/run workout, stretch and refuel before the swim.
	Run:		10-minute T-run	Z1		
	Swim:		10 to 15 minutes, laps or drills	Z1		
DAY 7	**Run:**		40 minutes	Z1		Typically, Day 7 will be your long run day. Keep it nice and easy as you head out today.

Olympic-Distance Training: Week 2

	COMPONENT			ZONE	REST	NOTES
DAY 1	**Swim:**	Warm-up	4×50	Z1	15 seconds	
		Workout	6×100	Z2	15 seconds	
		Cooldown	4×50	Z1	15 seconds	
		TOTAL	1,000			
DAY 2	**Run:**		35 minutes	Z1 or Z2		
DAY 3	**Bike:**		40 minutes	Z2 or Z3		Try to incorporate some hills on your bike. Start the run immediately after your ride.
	Run:		10-minute T-run	Z1		
DAY 4	**Swim:**	Warm-up	5×50	Z1	15 seconds	Incorporate at least three drills during your warm-up.
		Workout	6×100	Z2	15 seconds	
		Cooldown	4×75	Z1	10 seconds	
		TOTAL	1,150			
DAY 5	**Rest**					
DAY 6	**Bike:**		70 minutes	Z1 or Z2		Try to incorporate transitions on your long bike days.
	Run:		10-minute T-run	Z1		
	Swim:	(optional)	10–15 minutes, laps or drills	Z1		
DAY 7	**Run:**		45 minutes	Z1 or Z2		

Olympic-Distance Training: Week 3

	COMPONENT			ZONE	REST	NOTES
DAY 1	**Swim:**	Warm-up	4×50	Z1	15 seconds	
		Workout	10×50	Z2	15 seconds	
			10×25	Z2	10 seconds	
		Cooldown	2×100	Z1	10 seconds	
		TOTAL	1,150			
DAY 2	**Run:**		35 minutes	Z2		Keep the pace steady and attack a few hills if you're feeling up to it.
DAY 3	**Bike:**	Warm-up	15 minutes	Z1		
		Workout	25 minutes of			
			5×3-minute intervals	Z2 to Z3	2 minutes	
		Cooldown	10 minutes	Z1		
	Run:	(optional)	10-minute T-run	Z1		
DAY 4	**Swim:**	Warm-up	6×50	Z1	15 seconds	Strong swimmer: Do 6×150 (no 100s) and decrease rest times by 5 seconds.
		Workout	2×150	Z2	15 seconds	
			3×100	Z2	10 seconds	
		Cooldown	4×50	Z1	10 seconds	
		TOTAL	1,100			
DAY 5	**Rest**					
DAY 6	**Bike:**		75 minutes	Z1 or Z2		Strong cyclist: Do 4×5 minute intervals in Z3 during the ride.
	Run:		15-minute T-run	Z1		
	Swim:	(optional)	15–30 minutes, drills or laps	Z1		
DAY 7	**Run:**		47 minutes	Z2		Strong runner: Include a few minutes of fartlek.

Olympic-Distance Training: Week 4

	COMPONENT			ZONE	REST	NOTES
DAY 1	**Swim:**	Warm-up	4×50	Z1	15 seconds	Strong swimmer: Add two sets of 100 to the workout.
		Workout	6×100	Z2	15 seconds	
		Cooldown	6×25	Z1	10 seconds	
		TOTAL	950			
DAY 2	**Run:**	Warm-up	10 minutes	Z1		Stay below Z4 when you're picking up the pace.
		Workout	15 minutes of fartlek	Z3		
			1×25 per leg of each drill			
		Cooldown	10 minutes	Z1		
DAY 3	**Bike:**		30 minutes	Z2		Think about your form. Keep your neck and shoulders relaxed.
DAY 4	**Swim:**	Warm-up	6×50	Z1	15 seconds	
		Workout	10×50	Z2	15 seconds	
		Cooldown	2×100	Z1	15 seconds	
		TOTAL	1,000			
DAY 5	**Rest**					
DAY 6	**Bike:**		60 minutes	Z1 or Z2		
	Run:		10-minute T-run	Z1		
DAY 7	**Run:**		35–40 minutes	Z2		

Olympic-Distance Training: Week 5

	COMPONENT			ZONE	REST	NOTES
DAY 1	**Swim:**	Warm-up	6×50	Z1	15 seconds	Begin your bike ride immediately after getting out of the water.
		Workout	2×100	Z2	15 seconds	
			3×200	Z2	25 seconds	
		Cooldown	2×100	Z1	10 seconds	
		TOTAL	1,300			
	Bike:		10-minute T-bike	Z1		
DAY 2	**Run:**	Warm-up	10–15 minutes	Z1		See how you feel with a bump in intensity. The workout should take about 30–35 minutes.
		Workout	10-minute tempo run	Z2 to Z3		
		Drills	1×25 per leg of each drill			
		Cooldown	10 minutes	Z1		
DAY 3	**Bike:**	Warm-up	15 minutes	Z1		Alternate bike: Do 4 minutes uphill, 2 minutes downhill, and repeat 3 times. Pace yourself and try not to let your heart rate get too high.
		Workout	4×30-second SLDs			
			2 minutes	Z1		
			5×2-minute LGDs	Z2	1 minute	
		Cooldown	10 minutes	Z1		
DAY 4	**Swim:**	Warm-up	3×100	Z1	15 seconds	Strong swimmer: Add 5 more 50s to the set (total of 15), and decrease the rest for the 100s to 10 seconds.
		Workout	10×50	Z3	10 seconds	
			5×100	Z3	15 seconds	
		Cooldown	4×50	Z1	10 seconds	
		TOTAL	1,500			
DAY 5	**Rest**					
DAY 6	**Bike:**		90 minutes	Z1 or Z2		
	Run:		15-minute T-run	Z1		
	Swim:	(optional)	10 minutes			
DAY 7	**Run:**		50–55 minutes	Z1 or Z2		

Olympic-Distance Training: Week 6

	COMPONENT			ZONE	REST	NOTES
DAY 1	**Swim:**	Warm-up	6×50	Z1	15 seconds	Strong swimmer: Add a 200 and decrease the rest for the 100s to 10 seconds.
		Workout	6×100	Z2	15 seconds	
			2×200	Z2	20 seconds	
		Cooldown	5×50	Z1	15 seconds	
		TOTAL	1,550			
DAY 2	**Run:**	Warm-up	10 minutes, 6 accelerations	Z1		Strong runner: Add 3 intervals.
		Workout	15-minute interval set	Z2 to Z3		
			2 minutes pickup,			
			1 minute easy			
		Drills	1×25 per leg of each drill			
		Cooldown	10 minutes	Z1		
DAY 3	**Bike:**	Warm-up	15 minutes	Z1		Strong cyclist: Do 4 additional SLDs (total of 10)
		Workout	6×30-second SLDs			Alternate bike: Do 4 minutes uphill, 2 minutes downhill, and repeat.
			2 minutes	Z1		
			5×2-minute LGDs	Z2	1 minute	
		Cooldown	10 minutes	Z1		
	Run:	(optional)	10-minute T-run	Z1		
DAY 4	**Swim:**	Warm-up	3×100	Z1	15 seconds	Strong swimmer: Add an extra 100 and an extra 200.
		Workout	8×50	Z3	10 seconds	
			5×100, descending pace	Z2 to Z3	15 seconds	
			2×200	Z2	20 seconds	
		Cooldown	2×100	Z1	10 second	
		TOTAL	1,800			
DAY 5	**Rest**					
DAY 6	**Bike:**		95 minutes	Z1 to Z2		Start your run immediately after you get off your bike. If you can, try some open-water swimming.
	Run:		15- to 20-minute T-run	Z1		
	Swim:	(optional)	10 to 15 minutes, drills or laps	Z1		
DAY 7	**Run:**		55 to 60 minutes	Z1 to Z2		

Olympic-Distance Training: Week 7

	COMPONENT			ZONE	REST	NOTES
DAY 1	**Swim:**	Warm-up	3×100	Z1	20 seconds	Strong swimmer: Add a 200 and decrease the rest time by 5 seconds.
		Workout	6×200	Z2	25 seconds	
		Cooldown	6×50	Z1	10 seconds	
		TOTAL	1,800			
	Bike:		15 to 20 minutes	Z2		
DAY 2	**Run:**	Warm-up	10-15 minutes, 4 accelerations	Z1		Strong runner: Add 2 to 3 pickups.
		Workout	15-minute interval set			
			3×3 minutes pickup, 2 minutes easy between	Z2 to Z3		
		Drills	2×20 per leg of each drill			
		Cooldown	10 minutes	Z1		
DAY 3	**Bike:**	Warm-up	10 minutes	Z1		Do intervals or hill repeats for the 25-minute workout.
		Workout	25 minutes	Z2 to Z3		
		Cooldown	10 minutes	Z1		
	Run:		10-minute T-run	Z1		
DAY 4	**Swim:**	Warm-up	2×100	Z1	15 seconds	Strong swimmer: Add an extra 100 and an extra 200.
		Workout	8×50	Z3	10 seconds	
			5×100, descending pace	Z2 to Z3	15 seconds	
			3×200	Z2	20 seconds	
		Cooldown	2×100	Z1	10 seconds	
		TOTAL	1,900			
DAY 5	**Rest**					
DAY 6	**Bike:**		105 minutes	Z1 or Z2		Start your run right after the bike ride.
	Run:		15- to 20-minute T-run	Z1		
	Swim:	(optional)	15 minutes, drills or laps	Z1		
DAY 7	**Run:**		65 minutes	Z1		

Olympic-Distance Training: Week 8

	COMPONENT			ZONE	REST	NOTES
DAY 1	**Swim:**	Warm-up	6×50	Z1	15 seconds	
		Workout	4×100	Z2	15 seconds	
			3×200	Z2	25 seconds	
		Cooldown	4×50	Z1	10 seconds	
		TOTAL	1,500			
DAY 2	**Run:**	Warm-up	10 minutes, 6 accelerations	Z1		Keep a steady pace for the tempo run, don't sprint.
		Workout	10-minute tempo run	Z2 to Z3		
		Drills	2×25 per leg of each drill			
		Cooldown	10 minutes	Z1		
DAY 3	**Bike:**	Warm-up	15 minutes	Z1		Strong cyclist: Increase interval length to 4 minutes and reduce recovery time to 1 minute.
		Workout	5x3 minutes pickup,	Z3		
			2 minutes easy between			
		Cooldown	10 minutes	Z1		
	Run:		7- to 10-minute T-run	Z1		
DAY 4	**Swim:**	Warm-up	3×100	Z1	15 seconds	Strong swimmer: Do 7×200 instead of 10×100. Keep rest at 15 seconds.
		Workout	10×100	Z2	15 seconds	
		Cooldown	4×50	Z1	10 seconds	
		TOTAL	1,500			
DAY 5	**Rest**					
DAY 6	**Bike:**		80 minutes	Z1 or Z2		Begin your run right after your ride. Keep tweaking your "transition area" until you get it right.
	Run:		10-minute T-run	Z1		
	Swim:	(optional)	15 minutes, drills or laps	Z1		
DAY 7	**Run:**		50 minutes	Z1		

Olympic-Distance Training: Week 9

	COMPONENT			ZONE	REST	NOTES
DAY 1	**Swim:**	Warm-up	3×100	Z1	15 seconds	Strong swimmer: Add a 300 and decrease the rest time by 5 seconds.
		Workout	5×300	Z2	30 seconds	
		Cooldown	6×50	Z1	10 seconds	
		TOTAL	2,100			
DAY 2	**Run:**	Warm-up	10 minutes, 6 accelerations	Z1		Strong runner: Increase pickups to 3 minutes with 60 seconds recovery time.
		Workout	8×2-minute intervals	Z3 to Z4	45 seconds	
		Drills	2×30 per leg of each drill			
		Cooldown	10 minutes	Z1		
DAY 3	**Bike:**	Warm-up	15 minutes	Z1		Alternate bike: Ride for 10 minutes in Z3 to Z4, recover for 5 minutes in Z1, and ride for another 10 minutes in Z3 to Z4.
		Workout	5×1-minute SGDs	Z3	1 minute	
			2×2-minutes LGDs	Z3	1 minute	
			5×1- minute SGDs	Z3 to Z4	1 minute	
		Cooldown	10 minutes	Z1		
	Run:	(optional)	10-minute T-run	Z1		
DAY 4	**Swim:**	Warm-up	4×100	Z1	15 seconds	Strong swimmer: Increase each set by 2 and try to make each consecutive rep within a given set faster.
		Workout	7×100	Z3	15 seconds	
			100	Z1	15 seconds	
			7×50	Z3	10 seconds	
			100	Z1	10 seconds	
			7×25, descending pace	Z4	5 seconds	
		Cooldown	400	Z1		
		TOTAL	2,225			
DAY 5	**Rest**					
DAY 6	**Bike:**		125 minutes	Z1 or Z2		
	Run:		15-minute T-run	Z1		
	Swim:		15 minutes, drills or laps	Z1		
DAY 7	**Run:**		70 to 75 minutes	Z2		

Olympic-Distance Training: Week 10

	COMPONENT			ZONE	REST	NOTES
DAY 1	**Swim:**	Warm-up	8×25	Z1	5 seconds	Strong swimmer: Add a fast 50 (Z3) between the 500s (500-50-500-50-500) and decrease the rest by 20 seconds.
		Workout	4×500	Z2	60 seconds	
		Cooldown	6×50	Z1	10 seconds	
		TOTAL	2,500			
DAY 2	**Run:**	Warm-up	10 minutes, 8 accelerations	Z1		Strong runner: Make your high intensity spurts last!
		Workout	30-minute fartlek	Z3 to Z4		
		Drills	2×30 per leg of each drill			
		Cooldown	10 minutes	Z1		
DAY 3	**Bike:**	Warm-up	15 minutes	Z1		Alternate bike: Do 4 minutes up hill, 2 minutes downhill, and repeat 8 times. Strong cyclist: Do 10 reps instead of 8 (indoor) or 2 extra hills (outdoor).
		Workout	1 minute LGDs			
			1 minute SGDs			
			1 minute SLDs			
			Repeat 8 times	Z3 to Z4	1 minute	
		Cooldown	10 minutes	Z1		
DAY 4	**Swim:**	Warm-up	3×100	Z1	15 seconds	Strong swimmer: Add an extra set of 75s to your workout.
		Workout	3×75	Z3 to Z4	15 seconds	
			1×250	Z2 to Z3	15 seconds	
			Repeat 4 times			
		Cooldown	300	Z1		
		TOTAL	2,500			
DAY 5	**Rest**					
DAY 6	**Bike:**		135 minutes	Z1 or Z2		Do your T-run immediately after biking. You can wait until later in the day to swim.
	Run:		15-minute T-run	Z1		
	Swim:		15 minutes	Z1		
DAY 7	**Run:**		80 minutes	Z2		

Olympic-Distance Training: Week 11

	COMPONENT			ZONE	REST	NOTES
DAY 1	**Swim:**	Warm-up	3×100	Z1	15 seconds	
		Workout	10×100	Z3	15 seconds	
			5×200	Z2	25 seconds	
		Cooldown	4×50	Z1	15 seconds	
		TOTAL	2,500			
DAY 2	**Run:**	Warm-up	10 minutes, 5 accelerations	Z1		Strong runner: make your second tempo run 20 minutes long
		Workout	2×15-minute tempo run	Z3	2 minutes	
		Drills	2×15 per leg of each drill			
		Cooldown	10 minutes	Z1		
DAY 3	**Bike:**	Warm-up	15 minutes	Z1		Strong cyclist: make the intervals 4 minutes instead of 3.
		Workout	8×3-minute intervals	Z3 to Z4	2 minutes	
		Cooldown	10 minutes	Z1		
	Run:	(optional)	10-minute T-run			
DAY 4	**Swim:**	Warm-up	5×100	Z1	15 seconds	
		Workout	16×50, descending speed	Z2 to Z4	10 seconds	
		Cooldown	6×100	Z1	10 seconds	
		TOTAL	1,900			
DAY 5	**Rest**					
DAY 6	**Bike:**		150 minutes	Z1 or Z2		
	Run:		20-minute T-run	Z1		
	Swim:	(optional)	20 minutes, drills or laps	Z1		
DAY 7	**Run:**		90 minutes	Z1		

Olympic-Distance Training: Week 12

	COMPONENT			ZONE	REST	NOTES
DAY 1	**Swim:**	Warm-up	2×100	Z1	15 seconds	Strong swimmer: Add two 200s to second set.
		Workout	5×100	Z2	15 seconds	
			5×200	Z2	25 seconds	
		Cooldown	4×50	Z1	15 seconds	
		TOTAL	1,900			
DAY 2	**Run:**	Warm-up	10 minutes, 5 accelerations	Z1		Strong runner: Do a 20-minute tempo run instead of fartlek.
		Workout	20 minutes of fartlek			
		Cooldown	10 minutes	Z1		
DAY 3	**Bike:**	Warm-up	15 minutes	Z1		Try to find some hills for your workout.
		Workout	30 minutes	Z2 to Z3		
		Cooldown	10 minutes	Z1		
DAY 4	**Swim:**		50 minutes	Z1 or Z2		
DAY 5	**Rest**					
DAY 6	**Bike:**		105 minutes	Z1 or Z2		
	Run:		15-minute T-run	Z1 or Z2		
	Swim:	(optional)	15 minutes, drills or laps	Z1		
DAY 7	**Run:**		70 minutes	Z1		

Olympic-Distance Training: Week 13

	COMPONENT			ZONE	REST	NOTES
DAY 1	**Swim:**	Warm-up	8×25	Z1	5 seconds	Strong swimmer: Add a fast 50 (Z3) between the 500s (500-50-500-50-500) and decrease the rest by 20 seconds.
		Workout	4×500	Z2	60 seconds	
		Cooldown	6×50	Z1	10 seconds	
		TOTAL	2,500			
DAY 2	**Run:**	Warm-up	10 minutes, 8 accelerations	Z1		
		Workout	30-minute fartlek	Z3 to Z4		
		Drills	2×30 per leg of each drill			
		Cooldown	10 minutes	Z1		
DAY 3	**Bike:**	Warm-up	15 minutes	Z1		Strong cyclist: Repeat 10 times instead of 8.
		Workout	1 minute LGDs			
			1 minute SGDs			
			1 minute SLDs			
			Repeat 8 times	Z3 to Z4	1 minute	
		Cooldown	10 minutes	Z1		
	Run:		10 minute T-run	Z1		
DAY 4	**Swim:**	Warm-up	4×100	Z1	15 seconds	Strong swimmer: Add an extra set of 75s.
		Workout	3×75	Z3 to Z4	15 seconds	
			1×250	Z2 to Z3	15 seconds	
			Repeat 4 times			
		Cooldown	300	Z1		
		TOTAL	2,525			
DAY 5	**Rest**					
DAY 6	**Bike:**		130 minutes	Z1 or Z2		Strong cyclist: Add another 10 to 15 minutes to your ride.
	Run:		20-minute T-run	Z1		
	Swim:	(optional)	15 minutes, drills or laps			
DAY 7	**Run:**		80 minutes	Z1		

Olympic-Distance Training: Week 14

	COMPONENT			ZONE	REST	NOTES
DAY 1	**Swim:**	Warm-up	3×100	Z1	15 seconds	If you've been lifting weights, now is the time to stop. You can start up again after your race.
		Workout	5×300	Z2	30 seconds	
		Cooldown	6×50	Z1	10 seconds	
		TOTAL	2,100			
	Bike:		10 minute T-bike	Z1		
DAY 2	**Run:**	Warm-up	10 minutes, 6 accelerations	Z1		Strong runner: Increase pickups to 3 minutes.
		Workout	12×2-minute intervals	Z3	60 seconds	
		Drills	2×30 per leg of each drill			
		Cooldown	10 minutes	Z1		
DAY 3	**Bike:**	Warm-up	15 minutes	Z1		Alternative bike: Do a 10-minute interval in Z3 to Z4, recover at Z1 for 5 minutes, and do another 10-minutes at Z3 to Z4.
		Workout	5×2-minute SGDs	Z3 to Z4	2 minutes	
			4×2-minute LGDs	Z3 to Z4	2 minutes	
			5×2-minute SGDs	Z3 to Z4	2 minutes	Strong cyclist: Add one drill to each set (indoor) or increase intervals and decrease recovery (outdoor).
		Cooldown	10 minutes	Z1		
	Run:	(optional)	10-minute T-run			
DAY 4	**Swim:**	Warm-up	4×100	Z1	15 seconds	Strong swimmer: Do 9 reps instead of 7 reps of each set.
		Workout	7×100	Z3	15 seconds	
			100	Z1	15 seconds	
			7×50	Z3	10 seconds	
			100	Z1	10 seconds	
			7×25, descending pace	Z4	5 seconds	
		Cooldown	400	Z1		
		TOTAL	2,225			
DAY 5	**Rest**					
DAY 6	**Bike:**		115 minutes	Z1 or Z2		Don't forget to stay hydrated.
	Run:		20-minute T-run	Z1		
	Swim:	(optional)	15 minutes	Z1		
DAY 7	**Run:**		70 minutes	Z2		Pay close attention to your form.

Olympic-Distance Training: Week 15

	COMPONENT			ZONE	REST	NOTES
DAY 1	**Swim:**	Warm-up	4×50	Z1	15 seconds	
		Workout	6×100	Z2 or Z3	15 seconds	
		Cooldown	6×50	Z1	10 seconds	
		TOTAL	1,100			
DAY 2	**Run:**	Warm-up	10 minutes	Z1		Do a moderate run of 40 minutes, or incorporate some fartlek and some drills. Try to stay below Z4 when you're picking up the pace.
		Workout	15 minutes, fartlek	Z3		
		Drills	1×25 per leg of each drill	Z3		
		Cooldown	10 minutes	Z1		
DAY 3	**Bike:**		55 minutes	Z2		Keep your pace consistent and be mindful of your cadence.
DAY 4	**Swim:**	Warm-up	6×50	Z1	15 seconds	
		Workout	6×100	Z2	15 seconds	
		Cooldown	3×100	Z1	15 seconds	
		TOTAL	1,200			
DAY 5	**Rest**					
DAY 6	**Bike:**		80 minutes	Z1 or Z2		
	Run:		15-minute T-run	Z1		
	Swim:	(optional)	20 minutes	Z1		
DAY 7	**Run:**		45 minutes	Z2		

Olympic-Distance Training: Week 16

	COMPONENT			ZONE	REST	NOTES
DAY 1	**Swim:**	Warm-up	2×100	Z1	15 seconds	Race week is finally here! Now you really decrease the durations.
		Workout	3×100	Z3	20 seconds	
			4×200	Z2	25 seconds	
		Cooldown	4×50	Z1	10 seconds	
		TOTAL	1,500			
DAY 2	**Run:**	Warm-up	10 minutes, 4 accelerations	Z1		
		Workout	6×30 seconds	Z3	1 minute	
		Drills	1×20 per leg of each drill			
		Cooldown	10 minutes			
DAY 3	**Bike:**	Warm-up	15 minutes	Z1		
		Workout	35 minutes	Z2 to Z4		
		Cooldown	10 minutes	Z1		
DAY 4	**Swim:**	Warm-up	2×100	Z1	15 seconds	
		Workout	1×200	Z2	15 seconds	
			2×100	Z2	15 seconds	
			3×75	Z3	15 seconds	
			4×50	Z3	15 seconds	
			5×25	Z4	15 seconds	
		Cooldown	5×50	Z1	10 seconds	
		TOTAL	1,500			
DAY 5	**Rest**					
DAY 6	**Swim:**		10 minutes	Z1		Short workouts of everything to get your muscles loose after your rest day. If possible, do your workouts where you'll be doing your race.
	Bike:		20 to 30 minutes	Z1		
	Run:		15 minutes	Z1		
DAY 7	**Race day!**					

Race Day

As your race approaches, it's important to keep a good head on your shoulders and relax. Although it might be hard at times, try not to get too stressed out about physical, mental, or logistical factors. Your training schedule will help you reach your physical peak at the optimal time. Your mental preparation will have you in the right mind-set. As far as logistics go, you can verify last-minute details to reduce stress and curb unforeseen issues. This part will guide you through race day step by step, so you're prepared to cross the finish line and have fun.

Pre-Race Preparation

As your race approaches, you will begin to cut back on your workouts. This is called tapering, and it is built into the training plans in this book. During the end of your training program, the duration of your workouts decreases, but the intensity remains high initially. When it comes time to taper, you experience a short phase of considerably reduced activity just before your race. This part of your program can last between 7 and 21 days, depending on your current level of fitness and the distance of your race.

The longer the distance of your race, the more important this concept of staying off your feet becomes. In a super-sprint TRI, you might be only out on the racecourse for 45 minutes or so. With a race of this length, cutting back during the week before your event might not have a serious impact on how you feel out on the course. If you're trying to conquer an Ironman, you could be out on the course for 17 hours. In that case, the more downtime you get during your taper the better; your body will be that much more ready for a hard and long day.

Nutrition

As the race approaches, stick to what you know works for you nutritionally. This is not the time to experiment and eat new foods. Be careful if you go out to eat and stay away from unfamiliar foods. You don't want to find yourself feeling off at the start of your race because of a meal that didn't agree with you.

In the days just before your race, nerves, psychological factors, or thirst might cause you to want to drink a lot of fluids. If that's the case, remember to drink a sports drink that contains electrolytes like sodium and potassium. If you drink only excessive amounts of water, you'll dilute the amount of sodium and potassium in your system, which could lead to hyponatremia. You might not feel it until you're in the thick of the race and you have a cramp that you just can't seem to shake.

Mental Preparation

Mental preparation is as important as physical preparation. If your mind isn't ready for the upcoming physical test, you could find yourself feeling unprepared and extremely anxious. But you've made it this far through your training, so you can relax, knowing you've put in good, quality work. Manage your expectations, especially as a new triathlete. Race day is a time to cash in on all that hard work. You'll be ready to go when the time comes.

Try to systematically run through the events that will occur, and make mental notes on those items of greatest concern. Work to picture the different parts of your race, as well as the days and then minutes leading up to the start. When those moments come in real time, hopefully you'll be more comfortable because you've already visualized your success. Preparing yourself for all the things that might go wrong will have you ready to face anything fate sends your way.

Race Day Strategy

To make this day go smoothly, treat it like a training day. Wake up with enough time to eat, check and load up your gear, use the restroom, and get to the racecourse at least an hour before your race starts (if the transition area has a closing time, get there one hour before that deadline).

When you arrive at the venue, a buzz will fill the air. Take it all in. It's okay to have butterflies in your stomach; that is normal. Remember: your goggles are going to keep the water out of your eyes; your bike is going to perform just like it has in training; your running shoes are fine. If you've adequately trained and followed the pre-race checklist later in this chapter, you will be ready for this.

Check-In

When you get to the race, your primary objectives are to check in, give your equipment a final once over, and get your body marked with your race number (this may be written on your arms and legs with marker or applied as a temporary tattoo). Some people choose to kill two birds with one stone and ride their bike over to the body marking area. This way, you can confirm that your tires are properly inflated and get a chance to run through your gears.

Race check-in may occur several days before the race, or hours just before the starting gun goes off. Depending on your race, don't expect to get in and out quickly. Be prepared to wait a while, and do your best to show up at off times that might have shorter lines.

Race Packet

When you check-in, you'll receive a race packet. The contents of this packet will vary by race, but it will likely include the following:

- Swim cap, typically colored or numbered based on your wave
- Timing chip to electronically monitor when you cross various points on the course
- Race bib to display your race number
- Sticker with your race number for your helmet
- Sticker or tag with your race number for your bike
- Loads of advertisements for other races and possibly free samples of different fitness nutrition products

Transition Setup and Final Check

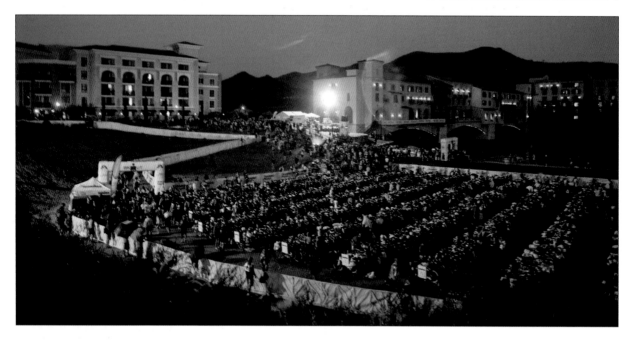

You should already have an idea about how to set up your transition area based on the transition workouts you did in training. The biggest difference is that you have to bring everything to your designated race transition spot and set it up there.

Find Your Spot

The transition area will have rows of bike racks that are usually numbered to correspond to participants' race numbers. When you find your assigned spot, double check that your bike tires are fully inflated and that you are in a very low (easy) gear.

If transition spots are not assigned by race number, you can lay claim to your territory by hooking your bike onto the horizontal rod in one of two ways:

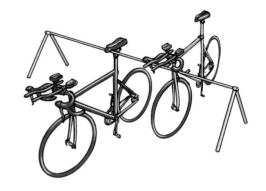

1. Hook the brakes of your handlebars over the rod.

2. Slide your rear tire and seat under the rod and then lift the front end of the seat and place it on the rod.

Get Organized

When your bike is secured, be sure the water bottles you plan to ride with are filled and in their cages (if you're using some other sort of hydration system, be sure it's filled and ready). Then spread out your transition towel on the ground next to your bike so you can lay out your other equipment. Decide where you're going to put any discarded swim equipment after you're done with the first leg of the triathlon, and leave a space on the towel or ground for those things.

Don't forget lubrication and sunscreen. Pull your clothing back several inches in any spot where it covers your arms and legs and apply sunscreen in those spots. That way if your jersey, shorts, or trisuit rides up during the race, your newly exposed skin will be protected.

In general, most TRIs follow a relatively standard set of rules. In the United States, USA Triathlon (USAT) is the governing body that dictates these rules. Even non-USAT-sanctioned races generally follow the same rules. Be sure you review the rules for your TRI, and ask questions of a race official when you're not sure about anything.

Warm Up

Unless you're doing a half-Ironman distance or greater, you should warm up your muscles and get the blood flowing about 20 minutes before your race starts. The easiest way to do this is to go for a short jog (no more than 10 minutes) or swim a few strokes. If there's no time to warm up before the start of your race, don't worry about it. Just be sure you start at a reasonable pace when the race begins. For half-Ironman distance or longer (which could take between 4 and 17 hours), you don't want to waste any of your energy stores by warming up. When the race starts, take it slow and ease into your pace. That will serve as the perfect warm-up.

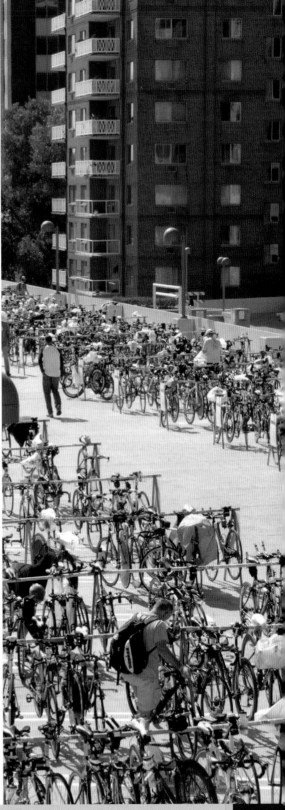

Swim to T1

Around 20 to 30 minutes prior to the start of the race, someone will start making announcements. Most race starts are separated into different "waves," which are groups of triathletes based on age, sex, and weight. The order in which the different waves begin can vary. Usually, you'll know prior to the race based on race paperwork you received. Get to the swim start on time.

Swimming will be the shortest segment of the race, both in distance and in time. However, swimming can be the scariest part of the day for someone who isn't mentally prepared for what's about to transpire. Don't panic! You will be prepared.

Find a spot in the water where you feel comfortable, don't worry about getting bumped by other swimmers, and remember that it's okay to take a break if you need it.

At the Start

The starting line may be in the water or on the beach. Wherever it is, find a spot in the crowd where you're comfortable. The fastest swimmers in any wave are always at the front of the group.

The start of the triathlon follows one of two methods: either everyone stands behind a line out of the water, or everyone is in the water behind a set of buoys or other markers. Either way, when the gun goes off, everyone heads for the most direct route to the first turn buoy. If you are in the ocean and have to force your way through any large waves, try to use the dolphin technique: simply dive beneath the large waves and come up after they've passed overhead. If the water is shallow enough to touch the bottom, use that sand to push off to return to the surface.

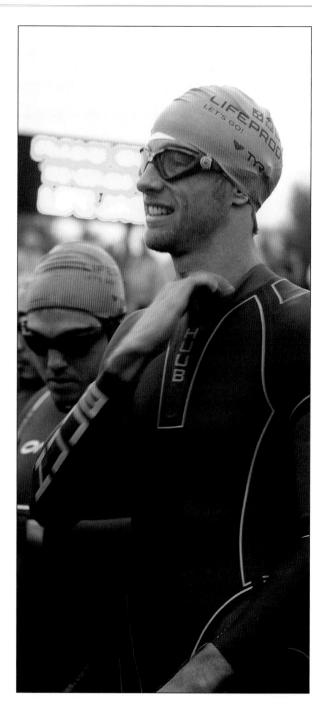

Positioning

Almost all triathlons start with the athletes in a pack and the champion swimmers positioned in the front of the group. If you weren't the captain of your swim team or are new to triathlon, position yourself wherever you feel most comfortable. If you're an average swimmer and feel relatively confident being close to other people in the water, move to the middle of the crowd. If you have some reservations about being around a lot of people in the water or you know you're a slow swimmer, try placing yourself near the back and on the far side of the bunch. Don't hesitate to go to the back or outside of the pack. The distance it will add to your race will be minimal, and it may make all the difference in your sanity.

In the Water

Your first few strokes may be lacking in form. You might not be able to extend your reach completely because someone's feet are in your face. You might not be able to pull correctly because someone is snuggled up next to you. When the madness of the start subsides and you get into your groove, run through this mental checklist of the form items you've worked on:

- Keep your chest down and butt up.
- Reach for it.
- Swim on your side.

Hopefully you've practiced siting while swimming in open water during training. Even though you'll likely have a crowd to follow in your race, don't forget to utilize this technique to make sure you're on track.

Before you know it, you'll be nearing shore and done with your swim. It will feel strange going from a horizontal position to a vertical one and running, but listen to your body as it adjusts, and go at your own pace. Find your transition area, and once there, use your head.

Two key things to remember during T1:

1. Be certain your helmet is on and securely latched.

2. Do not mount your bike until you are out of the transition area and past the mount/ dismount line.

If you fail to do either of these, you may be penalized or disqualified.

Bike to T2

Although there will likely be a crowd cheering you on right out of transition, be sure you don't go out like a rocket. Start off slow. Gradually increase your intensity until you reach your race pace and RPM range of 80 to 100. Going out too hard will cause lactic acid to begin to flow, so stay aerobic. Becoming anaerobic requires a period of metabolic recovery, which reduces efficiency and quickly depletes glycogen stores. Especially in the longer races, you don't want to fade during the final miles of the bike course. Pacing is the key; have patience and enjoy the ride.

Proper gearing is essential to maintaining pace and maximizing efficiency. Remember what you learned in training. Shift as often as necessary to leverage the chain rings for maximum efficiency. Gearing is individual to each triathlete's abilities, as well as to the topography of each racecourse. Remember that this is your race. Don't try to mirror other athletes' gearing choices.

After a couple miles in the saddle, your muscles might feel tight, so it's good practice to stretch out your body. Stand up from time to time and give your back a break. You can also sit tall and roll your neck and head. While stretching, be sure to keep your eyes on the road and stay in control of your bike. In addition to these strategies, remember to ride with a quiet upper body and loose fingers. Stay relaxed and conserve energy. Activate only the muscles needed.

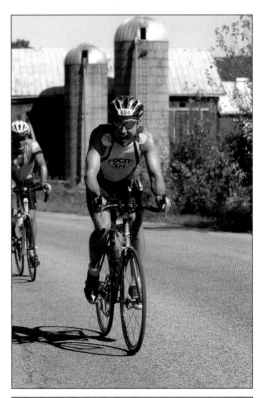

If there are aid stations (food and drink) out on the course, utilize them as necessary. Try to keep with the training regimen you have been using.

When you get to the end of the bike course, you'll have a sense of accomplishment and relief as you dismount the bike in the marked zone to enter the second transition (T2). If your bike shoes do not have rubber soles, be careful of your footing as you run into T2. Take your time and walk if you have to; a few seconds more in transition won't seriously impact your time.

Find your equipment, rack your bike, and swap out your bike gear with your running stuff (shoes, socks, hat, race-number belt, running belt, gels/bars, change of clothes, etc.).

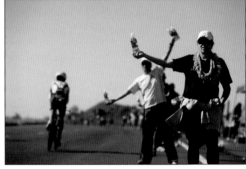

Run and Finish

The first few steps on the run course typically feel awkward. That feeling might last awhile, but be patient and let your legs switch from bike mode to run mode. Your training transition runs will show their value here.

Watch your pace, especially at the beginning. Don't allow the crowds and adrenaline to push you faster than your intended speed. Just as when you are coming out of T1, you want to stay aerobic. The goal on the run is to get from point A to point B in a smooth, balanced, relaxed fashion and to get there efficiently. Aim for comfort and remember good form. Focus so that your energy is channeled to contribute to forward movement, and keep your shoulders, jaw, and arms relaxed.

Remember and repeat these running concepts in your head:

- Stand tall.
- Just breathe.
- Don't bounce.
- Keep a quick cadence.
- Run relaxed.
- Land on your forefoot.

If you're struggling mentally on the run, try to break the distance into shorter segments by getting to the next tree, or the next mile marker, or the next aid station. Some people divide up their run into 10-minute segments, regardless of the distance (run 10 minutes, walk 1 minute). Whatever has worked for you in training will continue to work for you here.

Eventually, you'll approach the finish. You'll notice the cheer of the crowd increasing. Have fun with it. There's no rush to cross the line.

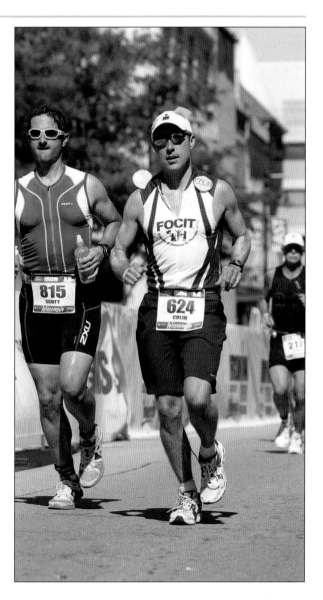

Fueling and Hydration

Eating a good breakfast or snack before the race will help you get through the swim. It is always a good idea to have a gel or other nutrition item with your transition gear for T1. After your nerves have settled and you've been in the water, hunger may set in. Better to have it there and not need it than the other way around.

If your race is long enough to warrant nutritional intake during the event, the bike segment is the best time to consume most of your calories. However, keep in mind that many triathletes need to allow their stomachs time to settle after a swim before eating. As a rule of thumb, "gradual is good." Again, do what worked for you in training.

It can be extremely difficult to grab food and drink from an aid station volunteer while on a bike. In your first attempt, you might drop that precious fuel because your momentum makes it difficult to hang onto the offered goodie. When rolling up to an aid station, slow down a bit. Then, reach for your item of choice, grab it, and let your arm sway back to absorb the impact. A stiff arm will most likely lead to a missed target.

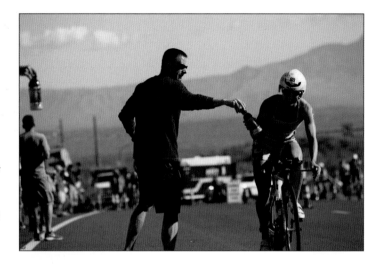

While out on the run (again, if the race length warrants it), you'll have to keep consuming calories. Continue to utilize the fuel you have with you, or items offered from aid stations to keep your energy up. Don't try anything new on race day and your digestive system will stay happy.

Especially in longer and hotter races, you must keep replenishing lost liquid and electrolytes throughout your day. You may need to walk to take a good drink, or you may choose to stop completely. Whatever works to keep your body hydrated and fueled is the right thing to do.

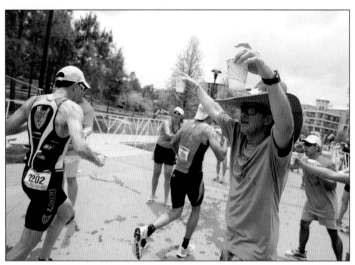

Race Etiquette and Tips

Be friendly and courteous while at the race venue, but especially before the race in the transition area. Many people will be stressed before the start of the race, trying to remember if they got every piece of equipment and arranging all their gear. Striking up a conversation might help you (and others) forget about your nerves, and a friendly acquaintance is less likely to squeeze in on your already-tight real estate. Additionally, if you later realize that you forgot something such as sunscreen or a floor pump, a good neighbor might be more willing to share his or her supplies with someone who has been kind. Just like in any other aspect of life, a smile and a friendly attitude will get you far.

During the race, you're going to pass other triathletes, and others will pass you. Realize beforehand that this is going to happen, and when it does, just let it happen. Let it go. The beginning of your triathlon career is no time to let your ego talk you into going too hard. Do the best you can, and don't worry about anyone else.

Stay focused on the given moment. Don't get ahead of yourself and don't think about the next phase of the race. In the present, you'll be most able to deal with a changing situation. Be prepared to pay attention to what's occurring around you. Focus on your intensity, know your nutrition plan, breathe, stay in the right rhythm, and make adjustments along the way.

Race Day Checklist

Don't wait until the day before race day to make a list of all the things you want to verify, and all the items you want to bring. Here's a sample race equipment checklist; you can use it as a base and adjust it based on your training experience. Some of the items are optional, and don't be afraid to add any additional items to the list. Utilize anything that's worked for you in training.

Swim

❏ Swimsuit or trisuit

❏ Wetsuit

❏ Wetsuit bag

❏ Swim cap (usually supplied)

❏ Goggles

❏ Defogging spray for goggles (optional)

❏ Earplugs and nose plugs (optional)

❏ Towel

❏ Supplies to rinse feet

Bike

❏ Bicycle

❏ Helmet

❏ Cycling shorts

❏ Jersey or singlet

❏ Bike shoes

❏ Socks

❏ Race wheels (optional)

❏ Pump, CO_2, and spare tube(s)

❏ Bike multi-tool

❏ Floor pump

❏ Duct tape and marker

❏ Chain lube (optional)

❏ Nutrition

❏ Water bottles and energy drinks

Run

- ❏ Shoes
- ❏ Socks
- ❏ Shorts
- ❏ Race outfit
- ❏ Race number
- ❏ Race belt (optional)

- ❏ Fuel belt (optional)
- ❏ Hat
- ❏ Sunglasses
- ❏ Lubrication
- ❏ Sunscreen
- ❏ Nutrition

Other

- ❏ Timing chip
- ❏ Eyeglasses or contacts
- ❏ Flashlight
- ❏ Toilet paper
- ❏ Towel(s)
- ❏ First-aid kit
- ❏ Heart rate monitor

- ❏ MP3 player
- ❏ Clothes (post race)
- ❏ Race checklist
- ❏ Race instructions
- ❏ Race maps
- ❏ Photo ID
- ❏ USA Triathlon membership card (if you're a member)

While you're checking things off your list, be sure to think about your travel plans. If you're traveling to another place for your race, confirm your travel arrangements at least a week ahead of time. Check your:

- Flight reservations
- Airline rules about oversized luggage (bike)
- Car rental reservations (Will the vehicle accommodate a bike or bike box?)
- Hotel reservations
- Weather reports

Prepare for the Unexpected

Most "unexpected" possibilities have been covered in other parts of this book. The two things you may not have encountered yet are the crowds and the nerves associated with a big event. The most important thing to remember at all times is not to panic. You will get through this.

Some people are struck with a feeling of sensory overload and nerves when they first arrive at their race—a feeling similar to stage fright. Prepare yourself for this possibility, especially if this is your first race. Everything will seem new. You'll question your training and your equipment. Just be prepared for this feeling and be ready to push it back into the depths. You are ready and your equipment is going to be fine. There may be butterflies, and that's okay. Remember that you are in control.

Swimming

Some triathletes experience a sudden feeling of claustrophobia during the swim event. This happens to triathletes of all levels, so don't be ashamed or think you need to pull yourself out of the race if it happens to you. If you feel that you're about to be struck by an anxiety attack, stop swimming, flip on to your back, and float or tread water for a bit. Move to the outside of the pack if you can. If not, don't worry. Look up at the sky and think about how much space there really is for you. Take a few deep breaths and just relax. Tell yourself you are prepared and you can get through this. When you feel that you've calmed down, start swimming again. Don't worry about any lost time.

Biking

On the bike, you'll be prepared for mechanical issues after all your training rides. The crowds will add obstacles, and if the race has referees enforcing a drafting rule, you might get "pulled over" for violating it. If this happens, try not to worry too much. Even the most elite triathletes lose concentration at times and drift too close to the bike in front of them.

Running

After swimming and biking at what might be a new intensity for you, the run may be tougher than you thought. You may have to reduce your pace from what you expected, and you may need to take in more fuel. Listen to your body, and push yourself as much as you can without risking a true injury.

Transitions

The transitions can cause some angst during a race. If you misunderstand the race layout and enter the transition area from an unexpected place, stop and try to figure out where your bike is based on whatever landmarks you can remember. If you get to the transition area and realize that you're missing something, you will most likely be okay without it. Make sure the item isn't hidden below your other gear, and then try to figure out if you should try to borrow from a neighbor, find it at an aid station, or go without it.

Safety Check

Proper lubrication and sun protection are two of the most important ways you can keep yourself safe. This should be second nature for you by the time race day comes along, but there is rarely a race that goes by where someone does not chafe a sensitive area or get a burn from the sun.

In all three disciplines, make sure to give other athletes ample warning and space when passing them. Especially during the swim, things will seem a bit frantic at times. Do not push, slap, or otherwise attack another triathlete. Remember, everyone feels just as crowded as you do at any given moment.

If you see a swimmer in trouble during the swim, it is your responsibility to let the lifeguards know. You might be the only one who notices their situation, so you need to act.

While on the bike, use the "on your left" announcement when you are ready to pass. During a race, there may be a very long line of bikers all looking to pass one another. If you don't let the biker ahead know you're coming, he or she might pull to the left at the same moment you are passing, causing a collision. Be courteous and aware.

If at any time you feel like you are having a medical emergency, stop and get help. Do not let pride take precedence over safety.

All that said, as long as you are smart and prepared, you will have a wonderful and safe race!

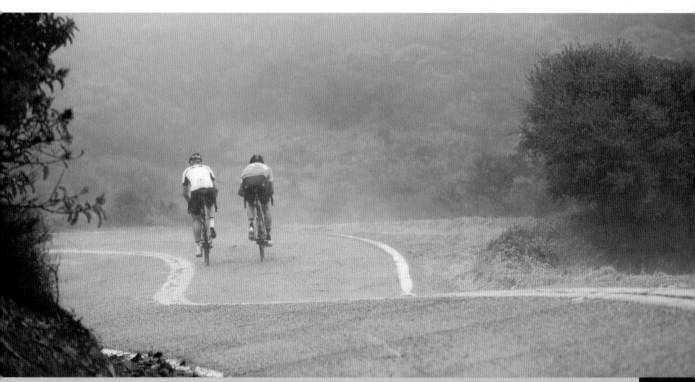

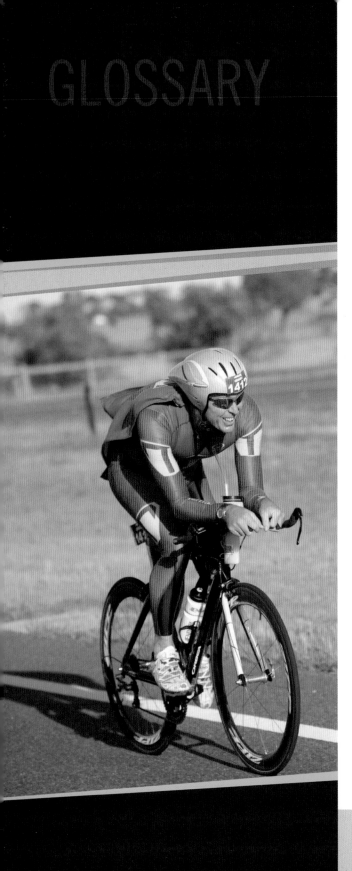

GLOSSARY

accelerations Starting with a slow jog, you accelerate continuously over a distance of about 100 meters until you're almost sprinting by the end.

active recovery Using exercise at lower levels of intensity to promote recovery.

aerobars A combination of handlebars and elbow supports on your bike that enable you to get your head and shoulders lower and more forward than you would be able to with regular handlebars. This position improves your overall aerodynamics and decreases stress on your back.

aid stations Volunteers set up at specific points throughout a race who offer athletes hydration/nutrition options (as well as moral support).

bike box A hard case used to pack a disassembled bike for easy transport or storage.

bike computer A tiny computer mounted on a bike, used to monitor data such as speed, distance, time, pedal rotations per minute, elevation change, etc.

bilateral breathing Alternating breaths between your left and right sides during swimming.

cadence The measure or beat of a specific movement (breathing, heart beat, pedaling, etc.). In cycling terminology, cadence refers to pedal revolutions per minute (RPM).

chain ring The front gearing of a bike. It's made of metal teeth that the chain sits on.

clincher tire A tire that "clinches" to the rim of a wheel. It tucks into the rim and is secured by the air pressure from the inner tube. This is the standard tire that is found on most recreational bicycles.

clipless pedals Pedals that lock to the cleat of a bike shoe (like a ski binding). Pedals of this type enable cyclists to generate maximum power in every rotation.

CO₂ cartridge   A small cylinder of compressed CO_2 that can be released through a regulator valve (adaptor) to inflate a tire.

cross-training   To attain fitness through more than one type of exercise.

descend   To complete several intervals of the same distance, with a decrease in time with each set.

drafting   To move close behind a moving object so as to take advantage of the slipstream (water or air). Drafting is illegal during the bike portion in almost all TRI races.

electrolytes   Nutrients required by cells to internally regulate hydration (sodium, potassium, etc.).

fartlek   Swedish for "speed play," a fartlek involves a warm-up and then a series of shorter, up-paced periods defined by distance between landmarks (city blocks), time, or general feel.

fatigue   The decreased capacity to function normally because of excessive stimulation or prolonged exertion.

fins   Swimming shoes that increase the surface area of the feet and enable the user to generate more power with each kick.

flexibility   The range of motion within a joint.

frame bag   A nylon box that sits on the top tube of your bicycle, behind the stem. It provides storage of things such as nutrition gels or bars.

frequency   The number of workouts performed in a given time frame.

hand paddles   Plastic paddles that strap to a swimmer's hands and enable the swimmer to generate more power with each stroke.

heart rate monitor   A combination chest strap and watch receiver. The monitor detects the heart rate and sends a signal to the watch receiver, which displays the heart rate.

hydration system   Any method an athlete uses to carry hydration fluids during activity, such as water bottles or backpack bladders.

indoor bike trainer   A device that allows any standard bicycle to become a stationary workout machine, with varying levels of resistance.

intensity   The stress level placed on the body.

interval   To work out with several periods of high intensity and a designated period of recovery. The periods are marked by distance or time.

kick board   A lightweight, foam board used to help keep the upper body afloat during swimming.

large gear drills (LGD)   A cycling drill performed using both legs in a large gear and a low RPM. These intervals are great for increasing muscular strength and endurance.

Master's Swim   An organized and coached workout with specific goals.

mount/dismount line   The boundary during a triathlon after which athletes can get onto their bike coming out of T1 or before which they need to get off their bike going into T2.

neutral roll   When, while running, you strike and then roll through the middle of the foot and off the middle or front section of the foot.

never-ending pool   A swimming apparatus that allows for stationary swimming with the use of a constant flow of water current.

overload   To push one's body to levels beyond a certain threshold (but below tolerance levels), to force beneficial adaptations that will occur in response to those demands.

overtraining   An advanced stage of fatigue caused from training beyond your body's ability to cope.

pace   The rate of speed at which an activity or movement proceeds.

presta valve   A long and skinny wheel air valve, usually used for road bikes.

pronation   When your foot strikes, rolls inward and forward, and then pushes off the ball of your foot or big toe.

pull buoy   A foam device you can squeeze between your legs during swimming to help lift your lower body.

race wheels   Nonstandard bicycle wheels used to improve aerodynamics.

rate of perceived exertion (RPE)   A scale developed by Dr. Gunnar Borg to measure one's subjective (based on feel) intensity.

repeats   A repetition of a specific distance or time within an interval.

rest   Recovery time taken after a period of increased effort, such as an interval.

reversibility   The decline of the body's fitness level after discontinuing a training program.

seat pack (saddlebag)   A general storage pouch hanging from a saddle or over the rear wheel of a bicycle.

set   A series of two or more repetitions of increased effort over a given distance or time.

shrader valve   Short and thick wheel air valve (like those on a car), usually used on bigger tires or older model bikes.

sighting   A technique used to keep on course while swimming in open water. The athlete simply looks for a landmark in the distance that's in the direction he or she wants to go and then tries to stay on that course.

single leg drills (SLD)   Cycling drills performed one leg at a time (with clipless pedals), in which only one leg is used to rotate the pedals at a time. SLDs are great for developing and improving the "full circle" mentality.

small gear drills (SGD)   Cycling drills performed using both legs with the chain in a very easy gear and high RPMs. These speed intervals help develop your neuromuscular system by teaching it to fire efficiently at higher rates.

Spinning   A group cycling class in which participants are instructed to vary their speed, resistance, and intensity throughout the workout.

static stretching   The preferred and most widely accepted method of stretching, which utilizes slow, gradual movements at low intensity.

supination   When a foot strikes the ground, rolls outward toward the outside of the foot, and then off the front-middle area of the foot/toes.

taper   The final days leading up to a race, when frequency, intensity, and duration are reduced to allow maximum rest and readiness.

target heart rate (THR)   The goal heart rate of a person participating in a fitness activity. (THR) = (220 − age) × desired intensity percent.

tempo run   After a warm-up, the tempo is increased to a faster-than-normal pace and sustained for the designated period of time.

toe clips   Plastic clips attached to the forward side of a pedal or pedal straps that help secure your feet to a pedal while cycling.

transition area   The area designated for changing clothing and gear when going from one sport to another in a triathlon race.

transition runs (T-runs)   A training run performed within minutes of the completion of a training ride. This helps prepare a triathlete's body for an actual race.

TRI-bag   A bag with specific compartments to organize TRI gear—shoes, helmet, wetsuit, etc.

tubular tire   One piece (tire and tube) that is wrapped around the wheel frame and inflated. Special wheel glue must be used to adhere the tire to the wheel.

wetsuit   A tight-fitting permeable suit worn in cold water to retain body heat.

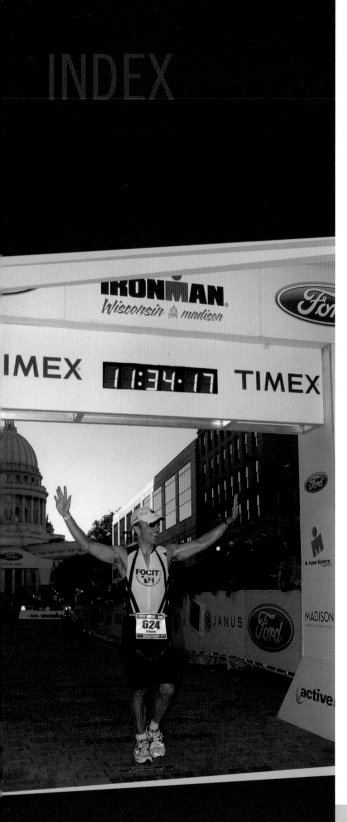

INDEX

H

Half-Ironman
  distances, 4
  training time, 14
Haller, Gordon, 5
hamstring exercises, 155, 177
handlebars for bikes, 30–31, 84–85
high knees, 123
history of triathlon, 5
hydration
  biking, 36–37
  hydration systems, 46
  running, 112–113
  running stage, 126
  T1 (swim to bike transition), 133

I–J

indoor training
  bike, 38, 96–97
  running, 116–117
injuries, 126
Ironman
  anniversary, 5
  distances, 4
  training time, 14

K

Katovsky, William, 5
kettlebells
  high plank row, 150
  swing, 157
kicking, swimming, 58

L

lateral lunge, 172
lateral raises, dumbbell, 168
LGDs (large gear drills), 97

location of races, 15
long races, 136
lubrication, 49, 77
lunges, 154, 159, 172
lying chest lift (cobra), 183

M

maintenance for bikes, 98–99
Master's Swim programs, 60
medicine ball, 153–154, 160, 166–167
mental aspects of running, 119
mental preparation, 226
mindset, 8
Moss, Julie, 5

N

night riding, 103
nutrition
  fueling during bike stage, 90–91
  nutrition belts, 46
  pre-race, 226
  race day, 234
  training programs, 195

O

Olympic, 4, 14, 17, 194–195
  week-by-week training, 208–223
Olympics debut of triathlon, 5
one-hand-on medicine ball push-up, 167
open water swimming versus pools, 60–61
  rip tide, 76
outdoor training
  biking, 92–95
  running, 114–115
overhead triceps rope stretch, 184
oxygen debt while swimming, 62

P–Q

P90X©, 7
pace, biking, 89
pacing, 16–17
packing
  bike leg, 102
  running leg, 112
Pan Am Games, 5
plank, 148
  kettlebell high plank row, 150
  side plank, suspended band, 149
PNF, 175
pools, 27
  versus open water swimming, 60–61
Presta valve, 99
pullovers, dumbbells, 169
push-ups
  one-hand-on medicine ball, 167
  two-hands-on medicine ball, 166

R

race day, 226–229, 234–239
rain riding, 103
recovery time
  Olympic, 17
  snacks, 113
  Sprint, 16
relationships, 8
rip tide in open water, 76
rows, kettlebell high plank row, 150
RPE (Rate of Perceived Exertion), 193
running belt, 47
running leg
  aid stations, 107, 113
  checklist, 237
  course layout, 107
  hydration, 126
  injuries, 126
  location, 107
  mental aspects, 233
  pacing, 233, 238
  packing for, 112

T2 (bike to run transition), 106
transition checklist, 138
weather, 126
running training
  accelerations, 125
  apparel, 44–45
  butt kicks, 122
  cadence, 109
  distances, 4
  drills, 122–125
  fartlek, 120
  form, 108
  fueling, 112–113
  high knees, 123
  hitting the ground, 110–111
  hydration, 112–113
  indoor training, 116–117
  intervals, 121
  mental aspect, 119
  neutral roll of the feet, 43
  outdoor training, 114–115
  posture, 108
  pronation of the feet, 43
  recovery snack, 113
  safety, 127
  shoes, 42–43
  side-stepping cross-overs, 124
  skipping, 125
  speed workouts, 120–121
  supination of the feet, 43
  technique, 108
  tempo runs, 120
  track, 118
  trail running, 115
  transition runs, 121
  treadmills for consistency, 116

S

saddle (bike), 83
safety
  bike leg, 102–103
  race day, 239
  running leg, 127
  strength training, 147
  swimming leg, 77
  transitions, 141

Photo Credits

Illustrations by John Fraser
2XU North America, LLC
    22, 38, 44, 45
Aqua Sphere
    21, 23, 24, 25, 26, 27
Event Photography Group, MarathonFoto™
    10, 85, 130, 133, 135, 232, 233
Gerard Brown © Dorling Kindersley
    28, 95
Mike Garland © Dorling Kindersley
    30
Philip Gatward © Dorling Kindersley
    41, 84
Grain Belt Pictures © Alamy
    57, 75
Noelle Katai
    7

Steve Katai
    32, 33, 35, 37, 39, 40, 42, 44, 45, 46, 47, 48, 96, 131, 136
Mark A. Lee © Alpha Books
    145, 146, 147, 148, 149, 150, 151, 152, 153, 154, 155, 156, 157, 158, 159, 160, 161, 162, 163, 164, 165, 166, 167, 168, 169, 170, 171, 172, 173, 174, 175, 176, 177, 178, 179, 180, 181, 182, 183, 184, 185, 186, 187, 188, 189, 191
Jay Prasuhn
    1, 4, 8, 9, 11, 12, 13, 36, 52, 53, 76, 80, 81, 86, 90, 91, 92, 93, 94, 102, 103, 106, 107, 113, 132, 134, 190, 230, 232, 240
Greg Perez © Alpha Books
    28, 29, 31, 34, 38, 39, 82
Russell Sadur © Dorling Kindersley
    7, 87, 115, 117, 118
James Tye © Dorling Kindersley
    62